ALSO BY DR. WANITA HOLMES

Stop Test Anxiety, Test-Taking Strategies that Use the Hidden Power of Your Subconscious Mind

Bar Exam Success, Use the Power of Your Subconscious Mind to Pass the Bar Exam

Sleep, Sleep, Sleep

Use the Power of Your Subconscious Mind to Sleep Smarter and End Insomnia in Just 21 Days

By Dr. Wanita Holmes

ISBN-13: 978-1519480828
ISBN-10: 1519480822

www.holmeshypnotherapy.com

The book you are holding in your hands will help you eliminate old thoughts and habits that have been keeping you from getting a natural good night's sleep.

This method works best when used with the companion Sleep Hypnosis MP3s available for purchase at:

www.holmeshypnotherapy.com/mp3s

TABLE OF CONTENTS

FOREWORD 1

YOU ARE NOT ALONE 3

DISCLAIMER 5

ABOUT YOUR MP3S 7

ALL ABOUT SLEEP 9

BEFORE YOU WERE BORN 9

THE IMPORTANCE OF SLEEP 10

WHY DO WE SLEEP? 12

WHY YOU CAN'T SLEEP 13

NO MAGIC PILLS FOR SLEEP 17

SLEEP PROBLEMS: YOURS, MINE, OTHERS' 19

WHAT IS YOUR SLEEP PROBLEM? 19

MY SLEEP PROBLEM 27

OTHER SLEEP PROBLEMS 35

TOO MUCH SLEEP, TOO LITTLE SLEEP 39

SLEEP CONFUSION, SLEEP SOLUTION 39

TO SLEEP OR NOT TO SLEEP 41

TOO MUCH SLEEP 42

TOO LITTLE SLEEP 43

BEAUTY SLEEP 46

SLEEP LOSS, FAT GAIN 47

21 NIGHTS 48

HOW HYPNOTHERAPY WORKS FOR SLEEP 49

RETRAIN YOUR BRAIN 49

HYPNOTHERAPY – IT WORKS! 51

DEMYSTIFYING HYPNOSIS..53

WHY YOU NEED TO LISTEN TO YOUR SLEEP HYPNOSIS
MP3 59

**SMALL BEHAVIOR CHANGES, HUGE SLEEP
RESULTS** 61

YOUR BED 61

HAVE FUN BUYING YOUR BED 64

S.O.S. HELP IS ON THE WAY 66

FAMILIES AND BEDS..69

CAFFEINE OR DREAM 75

DINE LATE, SMALL PLATE 79

GOOD FOOD HABITS FOR SLEEP 84

YOUR CLOCK IS YOUR ENEMY....................................87

EXERCISE YOURSELF TO SLEEP...................................92

BEDTIME READING...94

LIGHT POLLUTION 95

BIG MOON, LITTLE SLEEP..99

LET THE SUNSHINE IN... 101

YOUR NEW NIGHTTIME RITUAL 103

SLEEP TRAINING FOR EVERY AGE.........................**105**

SLEEP FOR ADULTS 105

SLEEP FOR SENIORS 107

SLEEP FOR TEENS 115

SLEEP FOR CHILDREN 119

SLEEP FOR SNORER AND SNOREE.............................. 123

COMMIT TO CHANGE..**131**

DEEP, DEEP BREATHS 131

PUTTING IT ALL TOGETHER....................................... 133

YOUR 21 DAY SLEEP JOURNAL **141**
    WEEK ONE 143
    WEEK TWO: 151
    WEEK THREE...159

ABOUT DR. WANITA.. **169**
    TESTIMONIALS..173
    CONTACT AND ORDERING INFO 177

FOREWORD

I have written this book and created the accompanying Sleep Hypnosis MP3s exactly the way I would if I were working with you as a private client in my office. Over the years I've realized that I can only see so many clients on any given day. I long to help many more people eliminate problems in every area of their lives, problems that are holding them back from achieving their goals and living their dreams. I have often thought, "How can I reach people who live far away or cannot afford to see me?"

My books and MP3s are the distillation of three decades helping people just like you. However, they are much more affordable than the $150 per hour to work with me in person!

This book is a friendly book, easy to read and understand. It is filled with information, simple explanations, and instructions that will enable you to get a good night's sleep.

I am sure that you have read or heard some of the information in this book before. However, this time I have kept it very simple to understand so that you don't let it go into one ear and out the other.

To get the most benefit from your book, I suggest you read it out loud. Read it several times.

That's right.

This will enable the information to go deep into your powerful subconscious mind. Using this information will make it easy for you to create new and powerful sleeping habits.

Get it: *You are what you think.*

Believe that you can sleep and you will sleep.

In order for you to get the most from your book I suggest that you purchase one of the companion Sleep Hypnosis MP3s I have created, which are available for purchase for a nominal fee at holmeshypnotherapy.com/mp3s

Then every night for the next 21 days, you will let your Sleep Hypnosis MP3 lull you gently to sleep. Just let the sound of my voice and the sound of the music slow down your brainwave patterns, easing you into deep, restful, peaceful, sleep.

Get ready for sleep.
Read this book.
Listen to your Sleep Hypnosis MP3.
Believe that you can sleep.
You will sleep!
Have a good night!

YOU ARE NOT ALONE

More than 70 million people in America are having trouble sleeping! Are you, or someone you know, one of them?

For many, many years I have been helping people learn how to create new and healthy sleeping habits. In this book I will tell you how I overcame my own sleeping problem. I promise to help you be able to get that longed-for, deep, restful, healthy, night's sleep, night, after night, after night.

Do you toss and turn for hours before finally going to sleep?

Do you go right to sleep and then wake up and can't go back to sleep?

Do you feel as though you never achieve a deep, restful, night's sleep?

Do you awaken in the morning tired and worn out?

If you are experiencing any of these problems with your sleep, then you need this book!

Disclaimer

This book will help you reach your natural ability to sleep. If you have a mental health or medical problem, please consult with a licensed health professional.

The information in this book and the accompanying Sleep Hypnosis MP3s are not a replacement for any treatment suggested by your doctor. Do not stop taking any prescribed medication without first discussing it with your doctor.

Warning: do not listen to any hypnosis recording while driving or using heavy equipment.

About Your MP3

This book has accompanying Sleep Hypnosis MP3s available for purchase at a nominal price on my website: holmeshypnotherapy.com/mp3s. The best way for you to get the quickest benefit from the information in this book is to purchase and listen to one of the hypnotic sleep MP3s I've created for you.

There are five different Sleep Hypnosis MP3s:

1. Adults or Seniors: *Sleep, Restful Sleep*
2. Teens or Pre-teens: *Lights Out*
3. Children (age 3-10): *Good Night Story*
4. Snorer: *Quiet Down*
5. Snoree: *Tune Out a Snorer*

Please pick the MP3 (or MP3s) that apply to you. You will use your MP3 only when you are ready to go to sleep.

Every night for the next 21 days you will listen to your Sleep Hypnosis MP3 and let it gently lull you to sleep. Just let the sound of my voice and the sound of music slow down your brainwave patterns, easing you into deep, restful, peaceful sleep. Get ready for sleep.

You must be committed to listen to your MP3 every night for 21 days until you have regained your new, natural sleep habit. **There is no need to force yourself to listen. Just lie back, relax, and let your Sleep Hypnosis MP3 put you to sleep.** Always remember that even when your conscious mind is sleeping and dreaming, your subconscious mind is still alert and listening to every word on your Sleep Hypnosis MP3, enabling you to reestablish your natural sleep cycle.

Listen to your MP3 every night for 21 days!
That's right!
Every single night!

If you should miss a night you must start all over again until you have listened for 21 consecutive nights. Remember, only listen to your MP3 at night when you ready for sleep.

Many of my clients tell me they continue to use their MP3 almost every night for years!

Your MP3 is very hypnotic and very powerful.

Never ever listen while driving!

To purchase, go to holmeshypnotherapy.com/mp3s

All About Sleep

Before You Were Born

You did not have to be taught how to sleep. Babies sleep in the womb.
That's right.
Think about that.

Sleep is natural.

There are three things that we never have to teach babies:

1. Fear of falling.
2. How to suck.
3. How to sleep.

Your problem is you have just *forgotten* how to sleep. I am going to help you remember how to sleep – deep, natural, peaceful, sleep.

You want to sleep or you would not be reading this book now. Together we will eradicate your old story, "I can't sleep," and create a new story:

"I can sleep."

Not only in the US, but also in the world, many millions of people are suffering from a catastrophic epidemic!

It is called "lack of sleep."

That's right. Just to name a few things, lack of sleep interferes with:

- Your health
- Your job
- Your schoolwork
- Your family
- Your relationships
- Your creativity
- Your thinking

In a large part of the world, people live in very stressful environments, which makes sleeping well more important than ever before. Always remember:

- Sleep is natural.
- Sleep is essential.
- Sleep is good for your mind and your body.
- Sleep is necessary to keep you alert.

A good night's sleep enables you to live a more relaxed, healthy and productive life, no matter what age you are.

This purpose of this book and your Sleep Hypnosis MP3 is to retrain your subconscious mind to remember how to sleep, to change your old story from, "I can't sleep, I am unable to sleep, I never sleep," to a new story: "I can sleep."

And then feel the magic begin to happen.

WHY DO WE SLEEP?

There has been much research done attempting to answer the question, "Why do we even need to sleep?"

There have been many attempts to answer that question. One thing we do know is that you need sleep to rest your brain and your body. Sleep restores your physical and your mental energy.

When you are awake your little three-pound brain is using one third of all your body's oxygen. The oxygen is carried to your brain from your blood flow. When you sleep, your blood flow slows down, which explains why your temperature goes down and you cool off at night.

We also know there is new evidence that sleep helps the brain to detox. That's right! Sleep enables the brain to wash away all the toxins that build up during your long hard day, toxins that are produced by your thinking. Researchers around the world now agree that this toxic waste removal system is one of the basic reasons for sleep.

How is your brain's cleaning system working?

Why You Can't Sleep

This book is really all about you. It is about changing the stories you tell yourself that cause you to be unable to sleep.

In early Roman times Cicero once said, "We often tell ourselves stories as though they were the truth even though we have never, ever, investigated them!"

Sound familiar?

I have been working with insomnia clients for many, many years and most of them have completely overcome their sleep problems. I tell my clients, "Not being able to sleep, is a habit, a habit you have created with the thoughts that you think. Since you have created the problem, you can uncreate it."

How? By creating new thoughts that you will be sending to your subconscious mind to change the way you think regarding your ability to sleep.

Sound simple? It is!

A very simple way to put it is this: **Your conscious mind thinks the thought and your subconscious mind acts it out.**

Whatever you tell your subconscious mind to do, it believes it is so and just acts on it. It's rather like your computer. Your computer 'believes' just what you put into it, hence the saying, "Garbage in, garbage out."

So when you say, "I can't sleep," that's garbage in. The subconscious mind now accepts the garbage as though it's the truth, which in turn affects your brain waves and creates chemicals in your brain and body to keep you awake, which now is 'garbage out.'

Always remember, your brain controls your body; your body does not control your brain.

Over and over during my sessions with my clients, they will declare with great emphasis, "Dr. Holmes, I *never* sleep!"

I tell them, "Of course you sleep. Maybe not the way you would choose to sleep, however you do sleep."

Others will declare,

"I am always tired!"
"I can only sleep when I take sleeping pills. I have become addicted to those damn pills."
"I hate nighttime. I dread going to bed."
"I am always cranky or edgy, because I am exhausted."
"Sleeping is impossible for me!"
"Sometime I want to just give up. Dr. Holmes, you are my last hope!"

Garbage in!
Is it any wonder that they can't sleep?

Many of my clients often treat their inability to sleep as the focal point of their identity. All their friends and family know every detail about their inability to sleep. I often ask my clients, "Who would you be if you were a sound sleeper?"

Then I say, "Listen, the more you talk about and ruminate about your sleeplessness, the more power you give it! Remember you are a body and thoughts and your thoughts always create your behavior. Therefore when you want to change a behavior, you must change the thoughts that are connected with that behavior. *Even if you don't believe those new thoughts,* the behavior changes almost automatically. Not sleeping is a learned behavior caused by your thoughts."

Over the years I have refined my knowledge and my understanding of sleep problems. I have to thank so many of my clients and so much of the available resources that have enabled me to develop many different ways to address sleep problems. Every day I work with problems that come from the mind (and what does not come from the mind?)

Decades of clinical experience have convinced me of the undeniable mind-body connection, and nothing responds more quickly or more easily to this mind-body connection than relearning how to sleep.

As you read your book, listen to your Sleep Hypnosis MP3, and make the suggested changes, you will soon learn to sleep well. You will wake up in the morning feeling rested, relaxed, refreshed and ready for the new day.

When you have read this book several times, and you have listened to your MP3s for 21 consecutive days, you will have learned how to change your story about your sleep.

Your sleep will improve.
Your disposition will improve.
Your wellbeing will improve.

Be ready to sleep every night.
Believe that it is so and it will be so!

You will get the results you want if you follow the instructions I will be giving you. Trust yourself!

Be open to believe that you can sleep.
Then relax and let it happen.
You will get a good night's sleep.

No Magic Pills for Sleep

Of the 70 to 90 million people just in the United States who have sleep problems, 9 to 10 million use prescription pills to try to get a goodnight's sleep.

How do sleeping pills actually benefit you?
They will enable you to fall asleep about 5 to 6 minutes faster and get 15 to 20 minutes more sleep.

Unfortunately most people often develop a dependence on sleeping pills even though they're not really getting much better sleep.

Now, what's the benefit for the pharmaceutical industries?

Big, big, money!

It is estimated that worldwide Big Pharma sells approximately $1.4 billion worth of sleeping pills each year. And they have been increasing their sales of pills every single year.

There are no magic sleeping pills! However there *is* magic in this book and your Sleep Hypnosis MP3. Remember, just a few changes in your subconscious mind can create magic. Simply be willing to be committed to do the work, be willing to make the changes, and then watch the magic begin to happen.
You can sleep.
You will sleep.

Sleep Problems: Yours, Mine, Others'

What Is Your Sleep Problem?

I assume that you purchased this book for yourself or because someone that you know has a sleep problem.

Right?
Okay!

We know there are several major sleep problems, which one is yours?

Do you toss and turn for hours on end only to find that you are absolutely unable to stop stressing out? Instead of sleep are you wide-awake, watching the clock as hours go by? Finally exhausted, you drift off in the wee hours of the morning.

Way too soon you are jolted awake by the loud, harsh sound of the alarm, or your kids, or your mate, or your pet jumping on the bed. You're not rested, just exhausted. You realize you need to get up and you need to get ready for the day. Just another day, tired, not rested, exhausted. You can't wait to get your caffeine fix so that you will have the energy that you need to help you to get moving.

Does this sound like your routine every day?

OR

Do you fall asleep easily after eating heavy meals late at night, perhaps drinking a few drinks of wine or a couple of martinis or several alcoholic beverages with your dinner? Do you get in bed shortly after you are finished eating your meal only to discover you are too tired for reading, TV, or even too tired for sex? You fall asleep soon after your head hits the pillow. And then you discover that night after night, at almost exactly the same time, you wake up and are unable to go back to sleep.

You lie awake and often you have to get up and take medicine for your acid reflux or heartburn from your undigested food. You are now wide-awake and uncomfortable. You wish morning would hurry up and come. When it finally does, you get up. It's just another day. You are tired, not rested, grumpy, exhausted.

OR

Maybe it is even worse for you. You have become addicted to either prescription or over-the-counter sleeping pills that leave you groggy and wiped out throughout the day. You go around declaring to yourself or to anyone that will listen, "I can't sleep!"

OR

Perhaps you are like some of my clients who get ready to go to bed every night, and may even look forward to a good night's sleep. You get into bed, turn off the lights, get yourself very comfortable, and then, suddenly you are WIDE AWAKE!

Just like that! Night after night, your brain begins to relive all the problems of the day. Have you ever noticed it's rarely reliving all the good things that happened that day? No, instead it is rehashing all the bad things, worrisome things, money problems, relationship problems, job problems, children problems, world problems, conspiracy problems, or your particular problem.

Sound familiar? You know what they are! Now you have created a real anxiety problem. You have created your "I can't sleep" problem, which has now become a habit.

Yes! Because now you are wide awake. You are very uncomfortable, hot, sweating, your nightgown, pajamas, T-shirt, or underwear is all in a twist. Once again, sleep has eluded you for yet another night.

All those worrisome thoughts that you are thinking are keeping you awake. These thoughts are interpreted by your subconscious mind as *real* so a flood of chemicals is released throughout your mind and body in response to your negative thoughts! Your powerful "I can't sleep" thoughts will keep you awake.

Every time you say, "I can't sleep, I never sleep, I hate going to bed, I dread the night," you are educating your subconscious mind to keep you awake!

That's right! You keep yourself awake. You have educated your subconscious mind day in and day out by filling it with all those negative thoughts that you can't sleep.

And so you can't.

Remember your subconscious mind does not know the difference between fantasy and reality.

Prove it?
Okay!

Why do you get scared while watching movies, so that you might actually hold your breath as you watch the Titanic sinking? Or you might get queasy watching Sandra Bullock has she floats and tumbles in space.

Is it real?
No!

It is just a picture on the screen. However your subconscious mind accepts that it's real so that you can experience the movie.

It is so very important for you to remember that the conscious mind thinks and then the subconscious mind acts.

What are you willing to do to help yourself get a good night's sleep?

Willingness is a state of mind. Be willing to be open and tell yourself over and over, "I used to have a problem sleeping, I choose not to have a sleep problem anymore."

Tell your subconscious mind, even if you don't quite believe it, that you deeply and completely believe that you can sleep. Tell yourself over and over again, "I am beginning to regain my ability to sleep because I am willing to do the work and change my thoughts to allow this to happen."

Have fun with this. Repeat it over and over when you are stuck in traffic. Make up a rap song. Sing it loud. Sing it strong! Be willing to do whatever works best for you to allow sleep to happen.

OR

Perhaps you are someone who gets into bed, arranges your body, your blanket and your pillows, you close your eyes and go right to sleep.

So far so good, but around the wee small hours of the morning, you are suddenly WIDE AWAKE and you can't go back to sleep. You check your clock and you know, just like all the nights before, it is always around the same hour. You know this because you always check your clock and then tell yourself, "Yep, right on time – again."

Irritated, you always get up, get yourself a drink, maybe go to the bathroom, maybe even smoke a cigarette, take a pill, and finally get back in bed, still wide awake.

You do this night after night. Understand this, you have been educating your subconscious mind that this is what it is supposed to do for you, to wake you up every night. And so it does exactly what you tell it to do. You have created a powerful **habit.**

How many times have you thought any of these thoughts or even said them out loud to yourself?

- "I can't sleep!"
- "I always awaken at the same time every night."
- "I can never go back to sleep once I wake up."
- "I will never ever get a good night's sleep again."
- "I always wake up tired and exhausted."
- "Why me? Other people sleep, why can't I?"
- "Dammit! I look at the clock and I want to throw it across the room!"
- "I dread nighttime. I give up!"

Let me ask you something. Have you ever had to get up early in the morning to catch an early flight when you are going on a vacation? You can't wait! You are so excited!

How many times have you missed your flight? Never? Wonderful!

That is because you are excited and have conditioned your subconscious mind to awaken you in time for you to get to the airport.

Many years ago I appeared on an early morning radio talk show. I had to be at the studio at 5:30 AM. I would set two alarm clocks, one by my bed and one in the bathroom. Not once did I ever need the alarm to wake me! On each occasion, I always woke up at 4 AM! I had conditioned my subconscious mind with my thoughts to awaken me at 4 AM, and it always did.

Get it!

Listen, this is important. You *must* stop telling yourself, "I can't sleep." You must stop telling yourself "I always wake up at the same time around three in the morning no matter what time I go to bed."

Instead, start telling yourself now, even if you don't believe it yet, "I can sleep. I used to be unable to sleep but I choose to sleep now."

Think about this, if you can keep yourself awake by the thoughts that you think, it follows that it is just as easy to tell your subconscious mind new thoughts that will put you to sleep.

So start telling yourself, "I can sleep. I choose to sleep."

Your subconscious mind doesn't care if you sleep or not, it simply does what you tell it to do. It will act on whatever information you give it. So read this book, follow the suggestions, and listen to your Sleep Hypnosis MP3 for the next 21 nights.

Go to sleep.
Stay asleep throughout the night.
Have sweet dreams.
Then continue telling your self, "I can sleep."

The great thing is you don't even have to believe it, not yet. Just say it! Say it over and over again.

Now, here is where the real magic begins. Even if you have to pretend for a while that your new way of sleeping is because of something that was done to you, and you really can't help it, your powerful subconscious mind begins to believe it and to do the work for you. Automatically.

You do have a choice. You can sleep. You are a sound sleeper. Remember, your thoughts create your reality. What thoughts do you need to change? Now is the time for you to change your thoughts about your ability to sleep. Begin to do the work, act as if it is so, and it will be so.

My Sleep Problem

I chose to write this book about sleep because for many years I've been helping people overcome their sleeping problems. I have worked with clients who have read many books on sleep, who have taken every kind of over-the-counter sleeping pill, who have tried prescription medicines, used herbs, acupuncture, alcohol, herbal tea, melatonin. You name it, they have tried it all – to no avail.

Recognize yourself?
Frustrating isn't it?

You already know that millions of people in America have sleep problems. They are all tired! You are not alone.

Just like you, I have had sleep problems in the past. Let me share with you exactly how that happened. When I was just 50 years old, I moved to Hawaii. Before that I never ever had any problems regarding sleep. My routine was always the same:

Get in bed.
Read a little.
Lights out.
Go to sleep.

Sounds great?
It was.

However, when I moved to Hawaii there was a three-hour time difference. In Los Angeles I always awoke at 6 AM without an alarm. I just woke up every day, seven days a week, year in and year out. Once I moved to Hawaii I began waking up every night at 3 AM. I would look at the clock and assure myself every time, "Yep, it is 3 o'clock here, that's 6 o'clock in L.A."

Night after night, year after year, for eight years I would wake up every night at 3 AM.

Then I began to tell myself I needed to get up and go to the bathroom. I would turn on the lights because I was afraid that I might step on a centipede, which are common in Hawaii, or maybe a cane spider, which are the size of a tarantula. Hawaii may be paradise but they do have scary bugs and I was always scared of stepping on one of them.

I would go to the bathroom, get a drink of water, get back in bed, and now I would be wide-awake. I would then need to read in order to relax and get back to sleep.

Sound familiar?

My story regarding my sleep problem was that at my age I probably had what many older people get, the need to get up every night to go to the bathroom. I would assure myself that this was a condition I had developed because of my age, and from now on my sleep would be interrupted night after night because I would need to go to the bathroom.

I also convinced myself that due to the three-hour difference in time between Los Angeles and Hawaii, that waking up at 3 AM in Hawaii was like waking up at 6 AM in Los Angeles.

All of this was just a story that I made up. A habit that I had created.

But then something happened! Eight years later I moved back to Los Angeles! What do you think happened in Los Angeles?

Maybe you guessed it, maybe not.

Even though I was in Los Angeles, once again at 3 AM I was wide-awake! Every night I would get up and go to the bathroom, drink some water and read for a while before turning off the light and going back to sleep.

Well, that blew my time-change story that I had created in Hawaii!

But this time something else had changed. I was now studying for my doctorate in hypnotherapy and I had started my hypnotherapy practice. I was busy learning all about the mind-body connection, about how the mind controls the body, not the body controlling the mind. I had learned how powerful our thoughts are, how powerful the stories we tell ourselves are, and how these thoughts and stories get stored in our subconscious mind and become habits that run our lives – for better or for worse.

One night shortly after moving back to Los Angeles I came home from a party around 1 o'clock. I put on my PJs, washed my face, brushed my teeth, went to the bathroom, and went to bed.

Lights out, no problem. I went right to sleep. It was about 1:30 AM.

At 3 o'clock, wide-awake.

What?

I told myself I needed to get up and go to the bathroom. I turned on the light. I got up. I went to the bathroom and while sitting on the john, I realized that just one and a half hours earlier I had gone to the bathroom, and here I was trying to go the bathroom again.

Yes! I had awakened at my usual 3 o'clock hour and had mindlessly gone into the bathroom.

Listen, my friends and family call me "camel bladder". I can work almost the whole day and never go to the bathroom. But that night after just one and a half hours, I was back up again at 3 AM to go to the bathroom. Conditioned to awaken at 3 AM, I simply woke up. Conditioned to go to the bathroom before going back to sleep, I went to the bathroom. No bladder infection, No bladder problems. I had just been training myself for eight years! I had educated my powerful subconscious mind, no matter what, to wake me up at 3 AM to go to the bathroom. I even kept my clock by my bed to reassure me that it was almost time to go to the bathroom, and no matter what I would get up.

I got it.

I had created a great story. I had created a powerful habit. Since I had created the habit I now would un-create it with hypnosis. I had been studying hypnotherapy and working with clients, so I decided to use hypnosis on myself to help me sleep through the night without interruption.

The very next night, the first thing I did was turn my clock around so that I couldn't see the time. After making sure I was comfortable, I began to do hypnosis on myself. I told myself I would sleep, deep, restful, continuous sleep. No need to awaken, just sleep, sleep, sleep.

Guess what!!
You probably guessed it. I woke up at 3 AM.

That's right!
But this time I told myself I would not get up. I told myself I would just take a few deep restful breaths and simply go back to sleep.

My bladder sphincter muscles were insistent!
Get up! Get up and go to the bathroom! Get up! However this time I did not get up. Instead I took a few more deep relaxing breaths.

The next thing I knew, I awoke and it was 6 AM. I had slept the night without getting up!

The following night I hypnotized myself before going to sleep, and once again I awakened to get up at 3 o'clock. Again I did not get up, even though my bladder was screaming at me, "I'm full! You need to empty me now! Get up."

Instead, I did some deep breathing, did more hypnosis on myself, and went right back to sleep. When I awoke it was 6 AM.

I felt empowered!

On the third night I slept throughout the night without waking. It was delicious, restful, peaceful, sleep. Today, except for rare occasions or having too much caffeine, I sleep peacefully and soundly throughout the night.

I did it! I had created the habit of waking up at 3 AM, and I uncreated it with hypnosis.
And so can you.

Many years passed until I was 82 and I developed my second sleep problem. My daughter and I were going to the theater one rainy night. All the marble around the entrance to the theater was very wet and slippery. We were walking very carefully but suddenly my feet went out from under me. I had my arm interlaced with her arm and we both went down. Everyone was amazed that at my age of 82 I did not break my hip. However I did suffer some trauma, which became arthritis and subsequently developed tremendous pain in my hip. Every time I moved in my bed at night, it would awaken me from a deep sleep. I could get maybe three hours of sleep at a time before I would be awakened yet again by the pain. I would then read for another couple of hours, fall asleep, then awaken again from the pain, and then I would just read until morning. I wasn't getting the rest I needed. I was working every day, using a wheel chair, exhausted, cranky, and refusing to take pain pills.

What is it they say? "Doctor, heal thyself." Once again I began to use hypnosis on myself every night and I started to get longer and more restful sleep.

Eventually, I had to have hip replacement surgery. It did the trick. I no longer use a wheelchair, nor do I need a cane. I am up and about, working every day, partying many nights, having fun, and sleeping great.

Please realize, dear reader, what happened to me regarding my sleep can happen to anyone. You and I can create bad sleep habits. When I applied the strategies I used to help others, they worked for me too. I slept easily and soundly.

That is why I decided to write this book and to make the same methods I use in my private practice available to millions of habitually tired people who cannot get to my office or cannot afford my fees.

This book is written as though I were working with you as a client in my office. It will change your "I cannot sleep" stories. It will eliminate your negative thoughts pertaining to sleep and will teach your subconscious mind to get rid of those self-destructive thoughts, thoughts that you had in the past that prevented you from having a good night's sleep.

Every night for 21 nights, you must listen to your MP3. Play it softly, allowing it to gently lull you to sleep.

Read and reread this book; read out loud, underline, highlight, dog-ear the pages – whatever enables you to get the messages you need to enable you to sleep.

Be committed to do the work and make the changes you needed in order for you to break your "I can't sleep" habit. Then, sooner than you think, maybe not as soon as you would have liked, you will have deep, restful, continuous, sleep.

I did it.
So can you.

OTHER SLEEP PROBLEMS

You are just one of the many people who have the same problem sleeping as you do. You simply are unable to get a decent, restful night's sleep. Many of the obvious reasons that can prevent one from getting the sleep they desire are listed below.

Please check off the ones that apply to you:

- o Apnea
- o Post-traumatic Stress Disorder (PTSD)
- o Nightmares
- o Night terrors
- o Snoring
- o Listening to a snorer
- o Noisy environments
- o Drugs
- o Alcohol
- o Smoking
- o Stress
- o Worrying
- o Eating late
- o Eating heavy, spicy, greasy dinners
- o TV
- o Computers
- o Mobile devices
- o Room too hot
- o Room too cold
- o Room too light

- Uncomfortable bed
- Restless partner
- Restless Leg Syndrome
- Caffeine
- Medication
- Full moon
- Daylight Savings time changes
- Kids in bed
- Pets in bed
- Anxiety
- Depression
- Medical problems
- Tension
- Boredom
- Overstimulation
- Pain

Do you recognize any of these sleep interference problems? How many apply to you?

Of course there are many more conditions or reasons (or thoughts) that can keep you awake. I wonder how many these conditions do you have? Many, or just a few?

It doesn't matter. You are going to make changes one night at a time. These problems will be addressed throughout this book. I know that many of the suggestions I will be giving you, you may have heard before. And that's okay. The difference is this time you choose to be committed to do the work needed.

Remember, "Success is the byproduct of work."

So... be willing to:

Follow the program.
Believe that it will work.
And then begin to look forward to many, many, good night's sleep.

Too Much Sleep, Too Little Sleep

Sleep Confusion, Sleep Solution

How many hours of sleep do you require? 4 hours? 6 hours? 8 hours? Nine hours? 10 or more hours? It's time for you to figure out how many hours of sleep you need to keep yourself healthy and rested.

In the past, research taught us that everyone needs eight hours of sleep. New studies have shown that belief was not based on fact.

The optimum numbers of hours for each age that I recommend are the following:

- **Adults** need about 7 hours of sleep.
- **Seniors** need 5 to 6 hours of sleep (and perhaps a nap during the day).
- **Teenagers and young children** need a minimum of 9 hours of sleep.
- **Babies** need 14 to 16 hours of sleep.

However the National Sleep Foundation released new guidelines in 2016:

- **Newborns (0-3 months)**: Sleep range narrowed to 14-17 hours each day (previously it was 12-18)
- **Infants (4-11 months):** Sleep range widened two hours to 12-15 hours (previously it was 14-15)
- **Toddlers (1-2 years):** Sleep range widened by one hour to 11-14 hours (previously it was 12-14)
- **Preschoolers (3-5):** Sleep range widened by one hour to 10-13 hours (previously it was 11-13)
- **School age children (6-13):** Sleep range widened by one hour to 9-11 hours (previously it was 10-11)
- **Teenagers (14-17):** Sleep range widened by one hour to 8-10 hours (previously it was 8.5-9.5)
- **Younger adults (18-25):** Sleep range is 7-9 hours (new age category)
- **Adults (26-64):** Sleep range did not change and remains 7-9 hours
- **Older adults (65+):** Sleep range is 7-8 hours (new age category)

And each one of these categories is not based on absolute facts!

Confusing isn't it? What is a person to do?

Keeping a Sleep Journal will help you determine the optimum number of hours for you. I will teach you how later in this book.

To Sleep or Not to Sleep

How many hours of sleep are just right for you? How much sleep do you think you really need? Keeping your Sleep Journal for 21 days will help you discover what's right for you.

Remember no one size fits all!

One thing we do know is that too much sleep is as harmful as too little sleep.

If you're an adult or senior, you no longer need to worry about getting eight hours or more of sleep. We now know that adults who consistently sleep 7 hours a night have the lowest percentage of premature deaths.

Too Much Sleep

Recent research has established that, for some adults, sleeping 9-10 hours or more, increases the risk of early death by at least 30%.

Adults who get 9 hours of sleep have the next highest premature death rate. Surprisingly, those adults who sleep 10 hours or more per night have a higher premature death rate than even those adults who sleep only 4 hours a night!

That's right, the adults who sleep 9 to 11 hours every night have the a premature death rate much greater than the people who sleep 4 to 5 hours, but not enough sleep causes problems too.

Too Little Sleep

Too little sleep is also bad for your health.

Inadequate sleep can make you more vulnerable for depression. Too little sleep can also cause high blood pressure, anxiety, weight gain, and predispose you to diabetes.

Too little sleep can be a killer.
Yes, You read that right.
A killer!

How many times have you heard or you have read about the tragedy when a train, bus, car, or truck causes an accident that kills or maims innocent people, all because someone fell asleep while operating a train, a bus, a truck, or a car!

There is also a tremendous loss of productivity due to tired workers. It is estimated that businesses lose over $20 billion a year because of errors, accidents, nap taking, and illness because of sleep deprivation. Being tired can even cause accidents that kill or injure people on the job.

The problem is most people are often unable to even recognize that they are tired. It is estimated that 20 to 30% of all fatal accidents are due to driving while sleepy! In a recent survey, 5% of California drivers admitted that at least on one day a week they have nodded off momentarily when driving while sleepy.

The question how much sleep do we need has plagued sleep experts worldwide. One British researcher argued that the brain needs only 4 to 5 hours of sleep. Dr. Daniel Dingus PhD later tested this assertion at the University of Pennsylvania School of Medicine.

Test subjects were allowed to sleep for only 6 hours each night. After only two weeks, one quarter of them were unable to keep from dozing off during the day. Additionally, some of the sleep-deprived test subjects performed as badly if not worse than if they were drunk!

This was a shocking revelation, as many train conductors, bus drivers, and long-haul truck drivers often get less than 6 hours of sleep.

We also now know that too little sleep is dangerous even for healthy people that who are allowed to sleep for 6 hours or less. Because of its effect on our hormonal production, inadequate sleep may cause us to be pre-diabetic, to age more quickly, to gain weight or to be depressed.

Scary isn't it?
It doesn't have to be.

Are you generally getting less than seven hours of sleep? Are you like one third of all adults in the US who are sleep-deprived on a daily basis? Are you using stimulants to get yourself through the day? Do you always wake up tired?

Then it's time for you to reset your own natural sleep cycle. How do you do this? It is simple!

You must plan on going to bed, and staying in bed, at the same time every night and awakening at the same time every day. This will begin to regulate your melatonin production and train your brain when to rest and when to be alert.

Remember each and every one of you has your own sleep requirements. It is time for you to discover what you need to do in order to be able to sleep soundly, peacefully and comfortably.

Be committed! Make the changes you need to make in order to improve your sleep habits.

You are going to change your sleep habits.
You can do it.
You will do it.
You are going to do it.

Ladies why do you think it's called **beauty sleep**?

They call it beauty sleep because when you sleep your skin begins to repair itself. If you don't get enough sleep, you will tend to look older much sooner than people who sleep well.

Research has shown that poor or inadequate sleep, (5 hours or less) causes people to have twice as many wrinkles, fine lines, dark spots, uneven pigmentation, and even reduced skin elasticity. However adults who sleep for 7 hours every night, who do not smoke, who always protect their skin with sunscreen, find that sleep is the very best medicine for keeping their skin healthy and radiant.

Sleep beats expensive face creams that sell for hundreds of dollars!

Sleep is cheap.
Seven hours of sleep!
That's it.
Sleep well.
The rewards are beautiful!

Sleep Loss, Fat Gain

Research now shows that sleep loss limits fat loss! Volunteers who were placed on a balanced diet for two weeks lost approximately 6 pounds during the two-week period when they had adequate sleep. 3 pounds of the weight-loss was fat and 3 pounds was lean body mass. During the two weeks, they slept an average of 7 hours a night.

When the same group slept only about 5 hours, and ate the same diet, over the same two-week period, they also lost 6 pounds but only 1 pound was fat the rest was 5 pounds of lean body.

Since we are a nation of sleep-deprived people, could part of our obesity problem be connected to a chronic lack of sleep?

Trying to lose weight while not sleeping well is doomed to failure.

Need to lose weight?
Learn to sleep great.

Remember, too much sleep *or* too little sleep can create health problems. Either one can increase the risk of diabetes, heart disease, stroke, weight gain, and depression. On the other hand, regularly getting 7 hours of sleep will protect most adults against many of the most common diseases.

So! Sleepyheads, for the next 3 weeks (that's 21 nights), be committed to reset your inner sleep time clock.

Read this book at least two times. Be sure to underline or highlight everything that applies to you.

Go to sleep listening to your Sleep Hypnosis MP3 every night at the same time, and wake up and get out of bed at the same time every morning.

Write in your Sleep Journal. (See instructions on page 141.)

Make as many changes as you need to make to enable you to find your natural sleep rhythm.

If you're an adult, start with your 7 hours. If you're a senior, start with 6 hours. Then stick with it! You will then discover that sleep is natural for you and you will learn you can do it!

21 nights to natural, deep, restful sleep.

How Hypnotherapy Works for Sleep

Retrain Your Brain

No matter what your reason may be for not sleeping, it will soon change. You will begin to sleep peacefully night after night. I have helped many people learn how to get a good night's sleep.

It isn't magic even though it may seem like magic to my clients. It is simply changing your thoughts and your attitude, regarding your sleep. As you retrain your brain over the next 21 days you will begin to erase all the negative thoughts that you have in your conscious mind. Thoughts like, "I can't sleep. I didn't sleep a wink last night. I never sleep. It's impossible for me to sleep."

You will stop these negative thoughts and stories and change them to new powerful thoughts and stories such as, "I used to be unable to sleep, however I now choose to sleep. I always sleep enough to awaken rested, refreshed, and ready for my new day!"

This is the good part: **You don't have to believe what you tell your subconscious mind.**

Just keep repeating to yourself, "I choose to sleep. I love to sleep. I can sleep. Sleeping is easy and natural for me." As you do this, your subconscious mind will hear these new powerful messages. Always remember, the subconscious mind does not know the difference between fantasy and reality, so it will begin to act as if it is true.

Repetition, coupled with commitment and determination will help you to achieve the healthy sleep habits that you long for.

Mark Twain once said, "There is nothing that training can't achieve." You are now beginning to train yourself how to sleep.

Sound simple?
It is simple.
Keep it simple.
Don't complicate it.

You have always known how to sleep. Never ever forget that no one had to teach you how to sleep in your mother's womb. You have simply forgotten how to sleep.

The information in this book and your Sleep Hypnosis MP3 will retrain your brain so you can enjoy sleep once again.

Trust yourself. You can do it.

Your reward will be deep, restful, continuous, healthy sleep.

Hypnotherapy – It Works!

When you have trouble sleeping, do you sometimes think, "I will never get a good night's sleep again?" Has your confidence to sleep simply disappeared over time?

Suspend your judgment!

Let go of your doubts *just long enough* to be open to some new ideas that will help you to sleep. Your thoughts can work for you, or your thoughts can work against you. Remember, when you want to change a behavior, you need to change the thoughts behind the behavior and then the behavior will change almost automatically. The way you focus on your sleep problem will affect your sleep.

One of the most powerful treatments for ending your sleep problem is hypnosis. How fortunate that you have this book to help you and your MP3 to listen to. If you haven't purchased your Sleep Hypnosis MP3, I strongly suggest you do so now!

Go to holmeshypnotherapy.com/mp3s to purchase your instant download.

Using both the information in this book and your Sleep Hypnosis MP3 will enable you to change the way you think about sleep and how you feel now about sleeping. With hypnosis, together we will change your subconscious thoughts and feelings regarding sleep and a new behavior will soon follow.

Results are typically seen within 7 to 21 days. My clients who have been willing to make the changes that are necessary have been very, very pleased with their results. Hypnosis works better than pills.

Are you committed to make the necessary changes, the changes needed to change your destructive bedtime habits?

Are you willing to:

- Use your bed only for Sleep or Sex?
- Go to bed at the same time every night?
- Wake up at the same time every morning?
- Read and review this book several times?
- Go to sleep every night as you listen to your Sleep Hypnosis MP3?

If you are willing to do these things, you will learn how to get a good night's sleep.

Be willing to make the changes. How does that feel?

DEMYSTIFYING HYPNOSIS

When someone new comes to my office, I always take time to explain what hypnosis is and how it works. This enables my client to be relaxed and to get the most from their session. I always record the hypnotherapy that I do with the client and then I give it to them so they can listen to it every night. Listening to their hypnotherapy recording every night enables them to make the changes that they choose to make in their life. Your MP3s will do the same for you.

I always ask the client about their ideas about hypnosis. I almost always get the same crazy, wild stories. The most repeated story is about someone who took off all their clothes and then danced naked in front of a large group of people and then when they were brought out of hypnosis they did not remember doing it.

Not possible! You are always in control when you are hypnotized. Not the hypnotherapist.

I want to share with you that in 30 years of doing hypnosis no one (that's right—*no one!*) has ever actually known the person who supposedly danced naked. It has always been someone who knew someone, who knew someone, who told the story. Furthermore, if this ever *did* happen, it would be because the person that danced naked really wanted to do it. Period!

Books, movies, and TV have provided us with erroneous ideas that the hypnotherapist takes over control of your mind and that they can make you do anything they want you to do! Not so! *You* are always in control when you are in hypnosis, not the hypnotherapist!

Hypnosis is simply deep, deep relaxation and a narrowing down of your focus. As you are reading this book you are in the "beta" state of consciousness. You are aware of your book, your surroundings, the sounds in the room, or the sounds outside the room. Your mind may even drift to something you need to think about, something you might need to do later.

In truth, while in beta you are not 100% focused. Your mind is busy, busy, busy, and this is as it should be. However, when you are relaxed in the hypnotic state called "alpha", you are very, very focused. All the chatter in your mind begins to slow down as you gently drift into the alpha state. Alpha is the way you feel as you begin to fall asleep at night. Not awake, not asleep, not dreaming, just relaxing and letting go.

When you enter into alpha you are in the healing place and the learning place. Everyone experiences alpha just before going to sleep at night and just before awakening in the morning, unless you are jarred awake by the rude sound of a loud alarm clock. This is called the hypnogogic state.

I always explain to my clients that I cannot make them do anything that they don't want to do. If I could, I probably would not be writing this book or perhaps not even working anymore. I would be rich – very rich – and the government would want me to hypnotize political leaders of other countries to do and to be the way our government wants them to be. Of course that is not going to happen.

When you are listening to your particular Sleep Hypnosis MP3, it will be working on your subconscious mind. Your subconscious mind is your best, most powerful friend. Your subconscious mind always does what you tell it to do. Remember your conscious mind thinks the thought and your subconscious mind acts it out.

Think of your conscious mind as the camera and your subconscious mind as the film. The film can only produce the picture you take. Remember your subconscious mind does not know the difference between fantasy and reality. Your subconscious mind does what *you* tell it to do. Simply put, the conscious mind thinks, the subconscious mind acts. You are what you think. You cannot escape it.

When you listen to your relaxing MP3 you will drift into a light, hypnotic, relaxed state. Your conscious mind will be resting while your subconscious mind is alert and listening. Only then does the critical censor in your conscious mind stop interfering with its "yeah but's, should have's, could have's and what if's."

Most people (maybe even you) have a complete misconception about hypnosis. They think they are under some kind of a mind control spell. My clients often ask nervously, "Are you going to put me under Dr. Wanita?"

"Under what? Under where? Underneath?" I ask them.

Then I smile and reassure them they're not going to be a zombie, or the walking dead, or feel like they are under anesthesia. I explain that they are not under anything. They are just relaxed. I then tell them you can hear when you are in hypnosis even though you may not hear consciously. Some clients, about 10%, hear every word I say on their MP3s. They are usually people in a position of authority, teachers, policemen, engineers, and control freaks! Your MP3s will work just fine even if you do hear every word that I say on your MP3s.

Another 20% say, "Dr. Wanita, I think that I heard everything you said." I tell them that's just fine. But when they come back for their second session they usually say, "Where the hell was I? I did not hear half of what you said on that recording!" I reassure them that they heard it all subconsciously.

Another 10% experience something called "audio amnesia." After I say about five sentences, their conscious mind stops paying attention. And that's just fine because their subconscious mind is focused and still listening.

The remaining percentage just goes tripping after hearing a few of my sentences. They just drift away. Some see colors, or hear music, some even work on another problem that they choose to work on. Then when my voice drifts back into their awareness, they think, "OMG she is still talking! I better listen!"

The truth is you don't have to *consciously* listen. Your subconscious mind is always listening. Remember whatever you choose to do will be just right for you. Trust yourself.

Even after explaining all of the ways one can experience hypnosis, some people still say, "I heard everything you said Dr. Wanita." I smile and tell them that's okay. Some say, "I think I was asleep." I tell them good, that's okay. Some tell me, "I didn't hear anything after the first few sentences," and once again I say that's okay. There is no right or wrong way to experience hypnosis. Just sit back or lie down, relax, listen to your MP3 and enjoy.

Always remember, hypnosis is natural. Research shows we go in and out of a trance state for a total of about two hours throughout every day.

Here are some examples:

- Sometimes while driving the same way to and from work every day.
- Sometimes when arriving at a destination and not remembering the drive there.

- Sometimes while doing a monotonous task over and over again.
- Sometimes while watching a movie and forgetting where you are.
- Sometimes listening to a long boring speech.
- Sometimes driving on a long trip at night on an open highway.
- Sometimes reading a book and getting so engrossed that you jump when the phone rings.
- Sometimes while doing stuff on the Internet, especially things like LinkedIn, Twitter, or Facebook.
- Sometimes while playing video games.

We have all done it!
It's natural.
It's just hypnosis.

WHY YOU NEED TO LISTEN TO YOUR SLEEP HYPNOSIS MP3

Ivan Pavlov, the great Russian scientist, taught us that it takes 21 days to create new habits, a new way of being, a new way of thinking. Pavlov used dog's to prove his point. Now, of course I know that you're not a dog, but still it takes 21 days – three weeks – to eliminate an old way of thinking and create a new way of thinking. Your sleep hypnosis MP3 will do this for you.

You will listen to them every night, let them put you to sleep, and while you are asleep and dreaming know that your subconscious mind is still alert, still listening, recording every word deep into your subconscious mind for you to draw upon each and every night.

Please note! Caution!

Do you not listen to your Sleep Hypnosis MP3 while driving or operating any moving vehicle, or while using any equipment that requires your full attention.

holmeshypnotherapy.com/mp3s

Stop!

If you haven't yet ordered your specific Sleep Hypnosis MP3, I recommend that you do it now.

Today!

holmeshypnotherapy.com/mp3s

SMALL BEHAVIOR CHANGES, HUGE SLEEP RESULTS

YOUR BED

One of the most neglected pieces of furniture in many people's homes is their bed.

How old is your bed?
How many times do you rotate your mattress?
How often do you wash your sheets?
How often do you air out your pillows and blankets in fresh air and sunshine?
How often do you replace your pillows, bedding, and blankets?

Be honest. Really think about this. You spend an enormous amount of time in your bed. Just look at the following accumulated hours you sleep per week and per year. You may be surprised by how many days you spend in your bed!

Highlight how many hours you sleep.

6 hours/night = 42 hours/week = 2,184 hours or 91 days per year.

7 hours/night = 49 hours/week = 2,548 hours or 106 days per year.

8 hours/night = 56 hours/week = 2,912 hours or 121 days per year.

9 hours = 63 hours/week = 3,276 hours or 136 days per year.

That is a lot of time in bed!

Get it, if you sleep 9 hours a night, you are spending about one third of your life sleeping in your bed.

We're not counting your tossing and turning, your waking up, or your being unable to go back to sleep, or all the other things that you do in your bed. No, we are just talking about the time you sleep!

It is time for you to wake up (no not from your sleep!) and begin to think about how much time you spend in bed. Realize that whenever you spend this much time doing *anything* you must pay attention to how you do it.

If you're anything like my clients, I would bet you've been sleeping in the same old bed for years, sleeping on the same old sheets, head resting on the same old smelly pillows, same old blankets, perhaps sleeping in a ratty T-shirt or an old nightgown, maybe baggy boxer shorts, or perhaps you sleep naked in an un-bathed body.

If I am right – and I usually am regarding this – it is time for a new bed, the very best and the most comfortable one you can afford. It's time for some new sweet-smelling pillows, new sheets, and soft comfortable blankets.

These simple actions can help you to look forward to getting in bed at night, to getting comfortable, and beginning to correct those old sleep habits as you tell yourself again and again, "I can sleep."

Do you think you cannot afford a new bed? Perhaps you can't afford *not* to get one. Start working toward that goal now. Every payday purchase one thing on this list:

- New pillows
- New sheets
- New blankets
- New bedspread
- New nightclothes

Next, turn your mattress over. If possible, air your bedding in the sunlight and the fresh air.

Every morning, make your bed.

Then take the next step. Start visiting stores that sell beds. Try them out. Choose a bed that you love. Do yourself a favor, start saving for your new bed now.

You need it.
You deserve it.

Have Fun Buying Your Bed

Your bed is ready to be replaced around every 7 to 8 years. That's right! How old is your bed? Some people sleep in the same old bed for an entire lifetime!

The idea of shopping for a new bed can be daunting and confusing. You're going to be like Goldilocks trying out one mattress after another, and like Goldilocks you will discover some beds that are too soft and some beds that are too hard. You likely will discover some mattresses labeled "hard" may really be too soft. Even more confusing, the same "soft" beds in one store might be labeled "firm" in another store!

You'll find spring coils, layers of foam, memory foam, different kinds of padding, pillow tops, adjustable beds, air-filled mattresses, water-filled mattresses, supportive mattresses, and last but not least, *comfortable* beds. So many choices!

But just as you would test drive a car, or try out a pair of new shoes to see if they fit, you are now going to do the same thing when purchasing your new bed.

A few things to remember:

Always start in the back of the mattress store. This is where the least expensive mattresses are displayed, price does not always equal comfort or durability. You may discover some real bargains.

Dress comfortably.
Be prepared to spend time in each store you visit.

Visit several stores, even if you wind up going back and purchasing your new bed from the first store you visited.

Take your time.
Enjoy yourself.
Don't be shy.
Ask questions.

Spend at least 10 to 15 minutes lying down on each mattress. Write down the names of the mattresses you try and request information or brochures regarding the mattress of your choice. You can then use this information you have gathered to compare the cost and the shipping fees for the same mattress online.

Important! Always ask about the return policy and how long you have to try out the mattress before being able to return it in case you're dissatisfied. **Get it in writing.**

Take your time. This is a 7 to 8 year purchase.
Watch for sales. Enjoy the process. Look forward to a good night's sleep on your new bed.

S.O.S. Help Is On the Way

S.O.S. The universal code for help!

For the next 21 days, your new, inviting, and comfortable bed is to be used *only* for sleep or sex, that's all.

Get it? Sleep or Sex! S.O.S.

Ladies, particularly single ladies, often do everything in bed *except* sleep – or sex!

They often:

Read and send e-mails.
Pay their bills.
Go online.
Check Facebook.
Browse LinkedIn
Tweet on Twitter.
Play solitaire.
Watch TV or movies.
Catch up on work from the office.
Eat.
Drink coffee, tea, wine, or alcohol.
Smoke a little dope.
Paint their toenails.
Text or call a friend.

Sound familiar?

No wonder your subconscious mind is totally confused! It thinks your bed is your workplace or your playpen.

Men are just as guilty.

They often:

Bring work home from the office and do it in bed.
Watch sports and get excited if their team wins or loses.
Play video games.
Watch porn.
Get horny and call a girlfriend or buddy.
Work on their laptop.
Drink a couple of beers.
Check email.
Cruise Facebook.
Go to an online dating service to see what's available.

Is it any wonder that your subconscious mind thinks your bed is for work or entertainment?

You have conditioned and trained your subconscious mind to believe your bed is your workplace or recreation room. Your subconscious mind no longer believes your bed is the place to rest, relax, and sleep.

Is this your S.O.S.?
Don't worry.
Help is on its way!

Sleep or sex, S.O.S. – that's it.
That is what your bed is for.

All you need to be is willing – willing to change your negative thoughts, willing to change your bad bedtime habits.

Are you willing?

21 days!

For the next 3 weeks, it's only S.O.S in your bed. Sex or sleep. And at the regular time you choose, listen to your Sleep Hypnosis MP3 as you fall asleep.

Only then can you easily and effortlessly create powerful new sleep habits.

Remember you have a choice. Will it be text or sex?

Read on.

FAMILIES AND BEDS

Parents, your bed is not to be used as a community gathering place. You have dens, living rooms, or kitchens for that purpose. Never forget, as an adult your bed should be used for only for S.O.S. Get it!

All too often several children wind up in the parents bed every night, where they eat in bed, fight with their siblings in bed, watch TV together do their homework, text on their phones, or play computer games. Many times they all fall asleep there and stay the night.

If this sounds familiar, it's high time to stop letting your bed be used as a free-for-all meeting place. Remember your bed is not a commune. Allowing children to congregate, or to fall asleep, in your bed will not help your child develop good sleeping habits.

It is time for you to teach your children that your bed is for you and their beds are for them. Give children the gift of enjoying a good night's sleep in their own bed.

Create nighttime rituals for your children. Prepare them for sleep by having them do several of the following at the same time, in the same order every evening:

- Take a bath
- Brush their teeth

- Put on their pajamas
- Go to the bathroom
- Get into bed
- Read them a short story
- Turn on a small nightlight
- Turn out other lights
- Kiss them good night
- Put on their *Good Night Story* Hypnosis MP3*
- Leave their bedroom door open

This will teach them that it is time for them to go to sleep in their bed, not in your bed. Your children will thank you later in life for helping them establish healthy sleep habits.

Remember your bed is where *you* sleep.
Enjoy it.
Sleep well!

*Available for purchase at
holmeshypnotherapy.com/mp3s

PETS AND BEDS

Your cat or your dog is your best friend!
But not in your bed!

Sleeping with your pet or pets is one of the most common causes of lost sleep. Over half of people who sleep with their animals admit their lovable animals disrupt their sleep. Yes, they are your friends, but they are your enemy in your bed. It is time for you to declare your bed a pet-free zone!

Pets can carry germs, germs that can cause dermatitis, cat scratch fever, and even staph infections. Yes, and they can even cause you to have allergies by leaving your bed sprinkled with their invisible dander. This dander can cause chest congestion, sinus problems, allergic reactions, breathing issues, and even snoring. All of these things can make it much more difficult to go to sleep, and to stay asleep.

If you are sleeping with your pet, it's time for you to declare that your bed is yours and it's no longer pet territory. Oh I know it's hard, my beloved Yorkie, Attila, used to sleep in my bed. But is it really hard? No, not very.

Interrupted sleep is hard! Lack of sleep is hard. Ask any parent of a newborn baby and they will tell you interrupted sleep is HARD and exhausting.

It is time for you to take charge of your territory. You have trained your pet that it is okay to sleep with you in your bed. Now, you will need to train your pet to sleep in a bed of its own. It will take some time, but it will be well worth it, even if you have to hire a dog whisperer, or a cat trainer.

Do whatever you need to do to reclaim your bed in order to get a good night's sleep. It will take some time.

It's worth it.
Do it!

BOOZE OR SNOOZE

When one of my clients reports that they easily fall asleep but awaken a few hours later, I ask them to answer the following questions:

Do you drink alcohol?
How much do you drink?
What do you drink?
How late at night do you drink?

Be honest with yourself. I would say 90% of my clients who have this particular sleep problem drink alcohol. They drink before dinner, during dinner, after dinner, and sometimes just before going to bed believing that alcohol will help them go to sleep.

These people are not necessarily alcoholics; they work hard, they need to unwind, and they have convinced themselves that alcohol relaxes them, and it does. But it also disrupts their sleep a few hours later. What fun is that?

If you use alcohol to fall asleep you are actually disrupting the brain's normal sleep cycle. That's right. You won't get the deep rest you need and you usually will awaken in the wee small hours in the morning.

Alcohol's effect on sleep is similar to sleeping pills. If you drink before bedtime you will discover you have a light, easily disturbed sleep, frequently awakening and finding it difficult to go back to sleep. You also may develop a dependency on alcohol to put you to sleep.

Also, drinkers often disturb the sleep of anyone else within earshot because alcohol relaxes your throat muscles, which can cause you to snore.

If you drink, you may need to begin to limit your alcohol. Ladies, have no more than one drink, and men no more than two drinks, 2 ½ to 3 hours before bedtime.

Start paying attention to how much and *when* you drink. Stop drinking at least 2 1/2 to 3 hours before bedtime.

Stop using booze to snooze.

I know that you may have heard all of this before.
This time get it!
You always have a choice.
Don't use alcohol to put yourself to sleep!

You can choose booze or you can choose to snooze. Which one do you choose?

CAFFEINE OR DREAM

To point out the obvious is no sign of my intelligence. Everybody knows that caffeine wakes you up. It makes you feel more alert and wide-awake. Brewing a delicious cup of coffee is usually the first thing we do in the morning to wake us up.

Unfortunately, most people drink coffee, sodas, tea, eat chocolate and other caffeine-loaded foods and beverages all day and often late into the evening, only to discover to their frustration that they can't sleep.

Caffeine is a stimulant, and it is the most popular stimulant in the world. Did you know that the caffeine in just one cup of coffee could remain in your brain and body for over 6 hours?

Rarely does anyone drink just a cup of coffee. Most of us drink 3 or more cups of coffee a day. We indulge in large cups of Starbucks, a cappuccino here, and a triple espresso there, and by the end of the day all that caffeine is still stimulating us and keeping us awake.

By the way, this does not include the caffeine we ingest in the form of medicines such as Excedrin, Anacin, diet supplements, cold and allergy medicines, and many prescription medications.

Is it any wonder that you can't sleep?

You do want to sleep or you wouldn't still be reading this book.

You must cut down or even eliminate your caffeine consumption. If you must, enjoy a cup of regular caffeinated coffee the first thing in the morning to get yourself going. For the rest of the day, switch to decaf. Make sure that the sodas you drink are caffeine free. Avoid chocolate desserts or candy late at night.

Read labels.
Say no to caffeine at night.
Sleep tight.
That's right.
Good night.

Cigarettes, Cigars, Nicotine

Are you like some of my clients who have a nightly ritual of smoking their last cigarette just before turning in for the night? Or if they should awaken during the night they reach for a cigarette on the nightstand and light up?

Do you believe like most of my stop smoking clients that cigarettes relax you?
They don't!

It is actually the deep inhaling of the smoke and then holding that smoke in your lungs, and then slowly exhaling the smoke that feels so relaxing. It's the deep breathing, not the smoke.

Nicotine is a stimulant. It is very similar to caffeine. It speeds up your brainwave patterns, constricts your circulatory system, which then elevates your blood pressure. Now your heart has to pump harder to circulate your blood. This produces cortisone, a damaging stress hormone.

Nicotine is a nerve poison.

Smoking irritates the mind and the body.
Smoking irritates your sinuses.
Smoking causes you to snore.
Smoking irritates your throat and your uvula.

If you smoke you will not be able to sleep well.
You absolutely will not be able to get a good restful night's sleep. In fact, insomnia is one of the major

complaints I hear from clients who come to see me for hypnosis to stop smoking.

It is time for you to get this!

Do you really want to acquire deep, restful, healthful sleep?

Do you want to fall asleep easily and effortlessly?

Do you want to stay asleep, and awaken at your normal wake up time?

You always have a choice.
You can choose smoking or sleeping.
Which do you choose?
It is really up to you.

DINE LATE, SMALL PLATE

I ask my sleep-deprived clients a very important question, "When do you sit down to eat your dinner?"

I am constantly amazed, even if they have children, how late many families sit down to dinner. More often than not it's between 8:00 and 9:00 PM.

Many years ago people ate a hardy breakfast, a hardy dinner at noon, and a very light supper in the evening. Conversely, today people now eat their largest and heaviest meal at night and often go to bed very soon after eating dinner.

Remember, when and what you eat has an absolute effect on the quality of your sleep.

I know you have probably read or heard this information before but this time I want you to really get it. **You need to allow 3 to 4 hours after you eat before you plan on going to sleep, or even lying down on your couch or bed.** Doing so will give you ample time to digest your food and avoid gastric reflux, which is when you burp up your food along with the acid that is in your stomach into your esophageal tract and sometimes even into your throat and mouth.

It's that nasty tasting, burning sensation that causes heartburn!

Heartburn can wake you up!

Heartburn and indigestion will keep you awake. You might even need to get up in the middle of the night to take heartburn medicine.

Whenever you eat a heavy meal, digesting all that food requires a great deal of energy and that will exhaust you! You work all day and stay up half the night, suffering from indigestion, heartburn, and discomfort, waking up to take an antacid.

Stop suffering night after night from gastric reflux. That is not enjoying living, that's just inhaling and exhaling and occupying space.

You deserve more. Be willing to commit now to change your habits. Be willing to change your life. Be willing to stop eating late or eating heavy meals before going to bed.

Your reward will be wonderful, uninterrupted, restful sleep.

No Pigging Out Before Bed

You now know that eating a large, heavy, greasy, or spicy meal just before going to bed can and will disrupt your sleep in many ways.

You now know you need about four hours after eating before you even lie down or think about going to bed. This will help you to not only sleep better but it will prevent food from being regurgitated into your esophagus and causing indigestion or heartburn.

But did you know there are foods you should always avoid as a late night snack just before "lights out"?

Highlight or check off all of the foods that you might eat late at night that will interfere with your sleep. Be honest.

Please don't read this list and skip highlighting. You are going to be reminding your subconscious mind which foods you should not eat so that you can get that good night's sleep you are entitled to.

- o Foods with MSG
- o Alcohol
- o Carbonated beverages
- o Coffee
- o Caffeinated tea
- o Fatty foods
- o Spicy foods
- o Garlic
- o Tomatoes

- Peppers (green, red, yellow)
- Beans
- Cucumbers
- Orange juice
- Candy
- Cake
- Ice cream
- Cookies
- Sweets or sugar (they can give you a burst of energy that can keep you awake.)

How many of these foods or drinks do you use as a snack before bed?

From now on if you get the munchies just before bed, try substituting a small carbohydrate snack, which will help you get to sleep. Eat a banana or a piece of toast. Sip some herbal chamomile tea. Try having a small bowl of sugarless cereal with low fat milk with a half of a banana.

Remember, you can eat in a way that will help you go to sleep. Complex carbohydrates will tend to make you feel sleepy. Complex carbohydrates increase your serotonin, a neurotransmitter that gives you a sense of peaceful wellbeing and helps you relax and feel sleepy.

Some research has shown that a small glass of warm milk will help put you to sleep, even if it is just the *thought* that produces the sleep.

We do know that our thoughts are powerful and magical.

What are your thoughts?

Change your thoughts and you will change your ability to sleep.

Change your habits and you will look forward to a goodnight's sleep.

Good Food Habits for Sleep

It has been found that having a serving of rice, pasta, potatoes, or whole-wheat macaroni with your evening meal will help you fall asleep much more quickly. These foods are but a few of the foods that produce tryptophan.

So for your dinner, three or four times a week and 3 to 4 hours before bedtime, eat some of those foods.

Most of you have heard that turkey contains tryptophan and eating too much of it at Thanksgiving or Christmas makes you sleepy.

Maybe so!

However studies have also shown that eating those large meals during the holidays requires a huge amount of energy to digest all that food.

That will make you sleepy, too!

It is true that turkey contains tryptophan. The question is whether it's the tryptophan or the digesting of large amounts of food that makes us sleepy? I suspect that it is a little of both.

There are some delicious snacks that you can eat just before lights out that will help you sleep.

For example, cherries. That's right cherries! An added benefit is that cherries have been shown to reduce or eliminate pain.

Just before bed eat one handful or one cup of fresh cherries, or 1/3 to 1/2 cup of dried cherries, or drink two tablespoons of cherry juice concentrate in one cup of water. This concentrate is equal to about forty cherries. Cherry concentrate can be purchased in any health food store.

OR!

You can just go bananas!

That's right. Eat a large banana just before bedtime and you will sleep like a baby.

Or you can eat any of the following tryptophan-rich foods:

- Avocados
- Hardboiled eggs
- Cottage cheese
- Yogurt
- Dates
- Hard cheese
- Milk
- Chickpeas
- Almonds
- Walnuts
- Turkey
- Plantains
- Chamomile tea
- Eggplant.

These particular foods will help you sleep. They also help produce serotonin, which helps you to relax so you can sleep.

It is important to note that certain carbohydrates can have the opposite effect:

- Candy
- Cookies
- Cake
- Ice cream
- Pie
- Sugar-coated cereals

The sugar "high" that you can get from these carbs will give you a burst of energy and keep you wide-awake.

From now on you must both:

Pay attention to *what* you eat at night AND
Pay attention to *when* you eat at night.

The rewards are worth it.
Peaceful, restful, sleep.

Zzzzzzzzzzz...

Your Clock Is Your Enemy

I wonder if you are doing exactly what I used to do. Do you wake up slightly in the middle of the night, force yourself to open your eyes and look at your clock to reassure yourself that you always wake up at your special time, every night?

Do you almost feel satisfied with yourself because you can count on the time that you awaken every night? It is always exactly or around the same time? Your trusty clock reassures you that you are right on target. Night after night.

Let me ask you something, have you ever had to awaken at a specific time for specific reason? Perhaps you needed to go to an early morning job interview or get to the airport very early to begin your vacation. How many planes have you ever missed when going on a vacation? Hmmmm?

Probably none! Why? Because you tell your subconscious mind that you want to get up at a certain time. What you tell your subconscious mind to do, your subconscious mind does. Most of the time you awaken even before the alarm goes off.

Right?
Yes!

You are up and you're ready to go. You feel delighted that you are in control, that you easily woke up when you needed to.

This is brain training.
Get it!

Remember the story I mentioned when had to wake up at 4 AM to make it to the early morning radio show used to do in L.A.? I would put an alarm clock on my nightstand, another one in the bathroom, and another one in the kitchen all set 10 minutes apart. Just in case. This was before snooze alarms!

Get this! Instead of telling yourself you can't sleep because you always wake up at the same time in the middle of the night, you are now going to change your story. It's just as easy to tell yourself you can sleep throughout the night until your normal wake up time.

First things first. Turn your clock or phone around so it's facing away from you. You don't need to see it during the night.

Tell yourself, "I will sleep throughout the night. If I awaken slightly I will not check on the time."

You can sleep until your normal wake up time.

Sounds too easy?
Sounds too simple?
Don't believe it?

Try it!
Then watch the magic begin to happen.

SOUND THE ALARM

Sleep is not the enemy.
The enemy is lack of sleep.

Did you know that when we change our clocks to daylight savings time we lose about 40 minutes of sleep? There is always a spike in workplace injuries and costly mistakes made during the first week of daylight savings time.

Loss of sleep causes people to make bad decisions, to cheat, to steal, and even waste valuable work time on the Internet doing personal stuff.

Arianna Huffington gets it. She fainted at work due to lack of sleep! She now tells all of her employees, "When you leave this office you are done working for the day."

You can feel the effects of getting just one good night's sleep almost immediately. So now you understand that you can actually sleep your way to success.

Google also gets it.
Google has installed sleep pads for employees to take naps. They know a well-rested employee works more efficiently and more safely.

MRI's show that a rested brain lights up in many areas while a tired brain hardly lights up at all.

Instead a tired brain will show that it is functioning in very few areas.

And yet many people think they are functioning well, when they are just sleeping four or five hours every night. They are simply kidding themselves.

Memory tests show repeatedly that sleep-deprived people do not function at their maximum capacity. Scientists know that chemicals produced during sleep help people repair their body and their brain.

One of the very important chemicals created when you are asleep and dreaming is acetylcholine. This neurotransmitter helps create memories and dreaming. When people have Alzheimer's, they stop producing much acetylcholine, their dreaming diminishes, and they begin to have memory loss. It is interesting that having vivid dreams is one of the side effects of Aricept, a common drug used to help Alzheimer patients! It would seem dreaming is beneficial for Alzheimer patients' brains.

Sleeping and dreaming are important for your mental health.
Sleep well.
Sweet dreams.

MEDS AND BEDS

Did you know that sleep is your best medicine?

Ironically not being able to sleep is often caused by the very medicine that you take. Have you ever asked your doctor or pharmacist if the medicine you're taking could interfere with your sleep? If the answer is yes, ask them if there is an alternative medicine that you could take, or perhaps you could start taking your medication in the morning or afternoon instead of at night. Many of my clients have found that simply changing their medicine or the time they take it has helped them to get a better night's sleep.

Medications such as blood pressure medicines, antidepressants, steroids, beta-blockers, pain pills, and many, many more may interfere with your ability to drift off to sleep.

Sleeping well balances your hormones, improves your immune system, helps keep your skin from wrinkling, balances your blood pressure, protects you from diabetes, and some new research indicates that deep restful sleep can increase your ability to lose weight. A good night's sleep is the greatest medicine that there is for you. There are no terrible side effects, just great benefits.

That's right! Just looking and feeling good.

EXERCISE YOURSELF TO SLEEP

Believe it or not, exercise will help you sleep better. Studies have shown that people who exercise for a minimum of 120 minutes a week are able to sleep much better. Here's the catch: Exercise will help you sleep but only if you stick with it.

You can walk on the treadmill, ride a stationary bike, or just go outside and take a walk for about 30 minutes. Do this at least four days every week. This will enable you to acquire about 60 minutes more sleep every night. That's even better than over-the-counter sleep medicines!

However, remember it takes discipline! You cannot just exercise for one day, or a few days, and then stop and expect a change in your sleep pattern. Sometimes it takes 2 to 3 months for you to be aware of the wonderful results.

Get it!
You need a 30 minutes of aerobic exercise at least 4 days per week for at least two to three months to get results to improve your sleep quality by 55 to 65 per cent.

Exercising will also decrease inflammation in your body. It will improve your metabolism. It will reduce daytime fatigue.

The question is what are you willing to do in order to get a restful, peaceful, relaxed night's sleep?

Are you willing to move your body for just 30 minutes 4 days a week? Are you committed to do whatever you need to do in order to quit feeling tired, cranky, depressed, irritable, and exhausted?

If you answered yes, get started now. Try it! Exercise 4 days a week. Feel how good you feel. You are now taking care of the place where you live: *Your body.*

You look better.
You feel better, and you sleep better!
How great is that?

If you feel that you must read in bed, read an *actual* book.

That's right. No electronic gadgets. No, Kindle, mobile phones, tablets or laptops. No! No! The blue light these devices emit will stimulate your brain to keep you awake. (See next chapter.)

Just read a paper book, an old-fashioned one with pages and printed words. Not an exciting or gripping novel either. Read a magazine, or a technical book, perhaps a book that you need to study for class.

Let your brain get weary; let your eyes get tired and begin to close. Maybe the book will fall out of your hands. GOOD!

When this happens, turn off the light, shut down your thoughts, count your blessings, and take a few deep, relaxing breaths.

Turn on your Sleep Hypnosis MP3.

Go to sleep.

LIGHT POLLUTION

Let there be less light!

It's not just teens, but most people who are suffering from the hours spent day and night staring at electronic equipment.

This blue light is very detrimental to getting a good, restful night's sleep. Exposure to any backlit electronic device is exposing you to blue light. Research has shown that this blue light suppresses melatonin, which makes it difficult for people to get to sleep easily.

Wearing orange, yellow or amber tinted glasses while using electronic devices will help to filter out this blue light radiation. Everyone needs to dim his or her electronic devices as much as possible, especially after sundown. This will help to lessen melatonin suppression.

This is a relatively simple solution. The hard part is to remembering to limit the time you spend using electronic devices, especially at night!

STOP!

Especially at night. You need to stop at least one hour before bedtime.

Yes, I understand, that this is not what most people want to do.

What? Give up using computers, Kindles, iPads, iPhones, TVs, Laptops?

If you are consistently using any of these electronic devices in the hours before bedtime, you will reduce your melatonin by the least 50%!

There is no dispute among experts regarding your constant exposure to electronic gear. Continued use will interferes with your sleep patterns and eventually will cause sleep disorders. Remember, lack of sleep often causes diseases so this is a health issue.

Some research indicates that people minimize the adverse health effects of blue light by sleeping in total darkness or using a small red light in the bedroom as a nightlight.

Many people around the world are suffering from too much light exposure, light pollution that causes them to feel mentally exhausted, irritated, depressed. This can lead to drug use, using sleeping medications at night, and using stimulants during the day to try to stay awake.

Immediately after the Northridge Earthquake in Southern California, people were calling 911 to report a strange phenomenon caused by the earthquake. They claimed there was a mysterious cloud hovering over Los Angles. It turned out to be the Milky Way that was now visible due to widespread power outages. Thousands of people living in cities around the world never see stars because of light pollution.

What? How sad that children can grow up to adulthood and never, ever have seen a heaven full of stars.

I grew up on Long Island, New York during World War II. Every night we had blackouts, which meant all shades drawn, all car lights covered with black tape, no street lights, no traffic lights, no houselights to be seen, only an occasional use of a flashlight.

But we had stars.

Every child could go outside and see millions of stars in the sky. We were connected to the sky, and space, and the planet, and the heavens.

I wish that today we could have a blackout at least one night a month in all cities, just for about 15 or 30 minutes, when the children could go outside and see what it is up there. It is truly beautiful!

Research has shown that too much nighttime light is messing with the sleep patterns of humans, and yes, even animals. All this light is causing sleep problems and risk factors for diabetes, cancer, heart problems, obesity, Alzheimer's disease, and even DNA repair.

Light pollution!
What is the solution?

- A dark bedroom.
- Don't use electronic equipment before bed.
- Blackout curtains.

These things will begin to protect you from light pollution. Try it for 21 days and you will feel the magic happening. You will look better, feel better, and last but not least, SLEEP BETTER!

BIG MOON, LITTLE SLEEP

The old song goes, "When the moon hits your eye like a big pizza pie, that's amore."

That's true! A big, beautiful full moon is great for love, but not for sleep.

Moonlight is not conducive for sleep; in fact it can make you toss and turn as its bright moonbeams light up your bedroom. If you are exposed to even a little moonlight during the night you will not experience deep restful sleep. And you may even awaken several times during the night and find it difficult to go back to sleep.

Several studies have shown that there is a downturn in sleep quality during the full moon phase. Many people experience losing any where from 20 to 30 minutes of sleep every night that the moon is full.

Even dim moonlight diminishes your melatonin levels, and you need melatonin to make you feel sleepy.

You need to do all that you choose to do to eliminate that loss of sleep. Make sure your room is dark. Invest in blackout curtains or buy some black material to drape over your blinds. Shut out those moonbeams.

Take a soothing bath before bed. Try sleeping with an eye mask. Spray some lavender essence in your bedroom.

Listen to your Sleep Hypnosis MP3. Let it lull you gently as the moon slowly sets and you go to sleep.

Sweet dreams.

Let The Sunshine In

Open up your curtains and your blinds and welcome as much natural light into your life as you can during the day. Before your morning coffee or tea, or your breakfast, let the sunshine in.

In order for you to have a good night's sleep you must, expose yourself to as much natural light as you can during the day. Believe it or not this will help you to get a goodnight's sleep.

Your mind and your body will gradually align itself to nature's rhythm. Daylight regulates the hormone melatonin, and remember, melatonin helps you fall asleep easier and sleep longer.

It is important for you to get adequate natural sunlight each day in order to sleep well. If you work in an office without windows you are only exposed to artificial light during your workday. Research has shown that if you work near windows that get natural light throughout the day, you will sleep 20 to 40 minutes longer at night than someone who works in a windowless office.

Have you ever stopped to think, why the highest paid workers, the CEOs, the presidents of corporations, always get the coveted offices where they have so many windows? It's healthier!

No windows?
No natural light during the day?
No good sleep.

If you have no windows at work, please go outside on your break times and take a short walk at your lunchtime.

Your mind and your body are geared to follow daylight and darkness. Start by getting as much natural light as you can during the day and as early in the day as you can. This will help set your body clock to be ready for sleep at night.

However always begin to avoid bright sunlight as evening approaches.

Remember it is not only the late evening news about murders, crimes, and terrorists that keep you from falling asleep. It is more often the bright glare of your large television screen that is keeping you awake because it suppresses melatonin production. If you must watch TV at night or be on your computer purchase amber colored glasses that will neutralize the blue light.

It's time for you to reset your mind and body clock.
You can do it.
It will help you sleep.

Your New Nighttime Ritual

It is important that you begin to develop nighttime rituals, which will alert your subconscious mind that you are now getting ready to go to sleep.

Here are some suggestions that you can begin to use every night as you are winding down and preparing to go to sleep.

Wash your hands and face because it just feels so good to feel clean.

Brush your teeth and as you brush them, pretend that you are brushing away all the day's problems, thoughts, and worries.

Have fun, and continue to imagine that as you clean your face and your hands and your teeth that you are cleaning up the day and getting ready for peaceful night's sleep.

Below are some other suggestions. Do any or all of these rituals and feel free to add you own.

The important thing is to always do the same things in the same way and at the same time, every night. This will indicate to your subconscious mind that now is the time for you to go to sleep.

- Get your coffee ready to go for the morning.
- Make the kid's lunches.

- Lock your doors and windows.
- Close your drapes or blinds.
- Turn out your lights in the house.
- Lay out your clothes and the children's clothes that are to be worn the next day.
- Spray lavender essence in your bedroom.
- Get in bed.
- Make yourself very comfortable.
- Turn on your Sleep Hypnosis MP3.
- Turn off your bedroom lights.

You really would rather sleep than stay awake, so remember these words:

Repetition, repetition, repetition!
Practice, practice, practice!

Do the same rituals every night and watch the magic begin to happen. You will sleep, deep, restful sleep.

Let it happen.

SLEEP TRAINING FOR EVERY AGE

SLEEP FOR ADULTS

As you've learned, depriving your brain of sleep not only makes you sleepy during the day, it also impairs your memory. It affects your ability to concentrate, your ability to perform complex tasks, and dulls your thinking.

A recent clinical study of thousands of adults from many different countries confirmed that 6 to 7 hours of sleep led to much sharper thinking. Too little sleep or too much sleep caused many in the study group to perform poorly on several types of testing.

If you're an adult, do your "3-pound universe", your brain, a favor. Commit to reestablishing your sleep cycle to be 7 to 8 hours of sleep.

- Go to bed at the same time.
- Wake up at the same time.
- Listen to your *Sleep, Restful Sleep* Hypnosis MP3 as you go to sleep.
- Keep a Sleep Journal (See page 141.)

Do all of the above 7 days a week for the next 21 days. Start with 7 hours then experiment with increasing your sleep time by 15-minute intervals, but sleep no longer than 8 hours.

As you practice the above instructions, you will find yourself feeling rested, relaxed, and more alert. Your memory and disposition will improve. You will then know that you have reached your perfect sleep cycle, the one that is just right for you. This will enable you to function at your highest level.

Make the changes.
Do the work.
It is not hard.

Going without sleep and feeling tired all the time is hard. All it takes is a little discipline and some commitment. You *will* get results.

After 21 consecutive days you will have educated your subconscious mind that sleeping 7 to 8 hours is natural. Now that you're learning how to do it, you can do it.

Enjoy!

SLEEP FOR SENIORS

Good sleep is the key to successful aging. Good sleep = Good Health.

More then half of people over age 65 have trouble falling asleep or staying asleep throughout the night. Older people often take long naps or go to sleep early in the evening only to awaken several times during the night. Sometimes poor sleep is caused by medications, or perhaps it's caused by a boring life-style with no exercise, too little sunshine, or too much loneliness. Sometimes the sleep problem is due to a physical problem, such as pain, or the need get up several times during the night to go to the bathroom.

The question is, do naps interfere with your sleep or do you need to nap because you do not sleep well? Many older people experience much lighter sleep and wake up more often during their night's sleep. This could be why they need to take a nap during the day.

Excessive worry can also interfere with a senior getting a good night's sleep. Some of the things seniors worry about include:

- Life
- Death
- Getting older
- Loneliness

- Family problems
- Medical problems
- Financial problems
- Boredom

Physical problems include:

- Hot flashes (for women)
- Low testosterone (for men)
- Sleep apnea
- Restless Leg Syndrome
- Muscle cramps
- Overweight
- Sedentary lifestyle
- Exercising too close to bedtime
- Eating too close to bedtime
- Caffeine
- Alcohol
- Snoring
- Dry mouth
- Low melatonin
- Medications

Seniors, how many of these things keep you awake? Check them off.

Research has taught us that older people often have reduced sleep needs as the required number of hours decreases as we age. The normal amount of sleep for those who are aging is about 5 to 7 hours of sleep every night, sometimes combined with a half hour nap in the early afternoon.

Now is the time for you to learn how to overcome your particular sleep problem. It is never too late to learn!

Exercise

Ideally, you should be getting at least 140 minutes of exercise during your week. That's equivalent to a bit more than 20 minutes of walking every day. This amount of exercise will help you to sleep better every night, to feel better physically, and to feel more mentally alert everyday.

Exercise reduces stress and exercise produces deep sleep at night. I recommended that you exercise in mid afternoon. According to experts, this is the very best time! Walk outside if you can. If not, try walking in place at home, perhaps while watching TV. Hold on to the back of a chair to balance yourself.

If you are disabled, roll your wheelchair back-and-forth or push your walker. It's important to move yourself physically anyway you can. Of course it's always a good idea to check with your doctor.

Sunshine

Normally, a melatonin surge happens as you begin to go to sleep; however this melatonin surge declines with age. This is just one of the many things that cause older people to have sleep problems. It is very important that you take time to get out in the sunshine every day in order to stimulate your body's natural production of melatonin and vitamin D.

Evening Lighting

Many older people get sleepy early in the evening. Unfortunately this causes them to often awaken very early in the morning. Light sleep seems to be more prevalent as adults age and, unfortunately, it is often thought to be a "normal" sign of ageing.

To prevent this from happening turn up your lights in the evening. Not bright lights! We've discussed how light pollution is detrimental to sleep. However, many older people choose to use only one small dim light at night to conserve electricity. This can cause them to get sleepy too early in the evening.

Instead, if it's early evening, turn on some lights and get up and move or do something to stimulate your mind:

- Do a task that you have been putting off.
- Have someone over for dinner.
- Do the dishes.
- Bake a cake.
- Do a crossword puzzle.
- Call a friend.
- Stay off the computer.

Connect with the World Around You

Sometimes not being able to sleep is a sign of depression and sometimes sleeping too much is also a sign of depression. Depression late in life can be a feeling of sadness due to a belief you're no longer able to enjoy pleasurable activities. Without a healthy social network, you can dwell too much on thoughts of the past. You may start worrying about the end of life, death, or even contemplate suicide. Any one of these things can be a red flag indicating depression. **If any of these apply to you please seek professional help!**

However there is a lot you can do to enjoy the present and connect with the world around you.

- Get socially involved.
- Visit a senior center.
- Go out in nature.
- Take a walk around the mall.
- Take up a hobby.
- Volunteer.
- Go to church.
- Read to children in your public library.
- Do something that makes you feel good, especially with other people.
- Adopt a pet.

No matter how old your mind and body may be, it does know when it's time for you to sleep. What you must do is establish a personal sleep ritual you perform every night, such as brushing your teeth, washing your face, brushing your hair, locking your door, getting comfortable in bed, listen to your *Sleep, Restful Sleep* Hypnosis MP3, lights out, relax, and go to sleep.

If you should awaken briefly during the night, just roll over and go back to sleep. Even if you need to get up to go to the bathroom, just get back in bed, make yourself very comfortable, turn your *Sleep, Restful Sleep* Hypnosis MP3 back on, and go back to sleep. Be sure to turn your clock to the wall! No need to condition yourself to check the time every night.

If you have a habit of awakening too early, choose to avoid bright lights or sunlight for a few hours after awakening. Also if you get tired before it is time for bed, once again, keep some bright lights on in the early evening.

These are problems anyone can have regarding their sleep. Both men and women at any age must create daytime and nighttime routines for better quality sleep.

Willingness is a state of mind.

Be honest with yourself. How many of the following are you willing to do?

Make the commitment and you will sleep.

- Read and study this book.
- Listen to your *Sleep, Restful Sleep* Hypnosis MP3. Studies have shown that hypnosis is extremely beneficial for sleep especially when combined with changes in your routine, your sleep environment, and ways of thinking about sleep.
- Go to sleep at the same time every night.
- Awaken and get out of bed at the same time every day.
- Get 20 to 30 minutes of exercise a minimum of 4 days a week.
- Get natural sunshine every day.
- No caffeinated beverages late in the day.
- No alcohol or cigarettes late in the day.
- Make sure you have great bed pillows, fresh blankets, sheets, and if needed, a new bed.
- Make sure your bedroom is a dark, quiet, cool room.
- Use your bed only for S.O.S. (Sleep or Sex)
- Keep a Sleep Journal so you can find your perfect sleep time. (See page 141.)

If you have trouble getting to sleep, get up, get busy, and do a small task you've been putting off. Don't worry too much about the number of hours you sleep; 5 to 6 hours is just fine for seniors when coupled with a half hour nap in the early afternoon.

If you doze off too many times during the day, or just feel tired all the time, talk to your doctor to rule out any health issues. Your doctor may refer you to a sleep specialist.

Simply be willing to make the changes that you need to make. Do the work you need to do to learn to sleep well.

Good night.

SLEEP FOR TEENS

At least 40% of teens between the ages of 12 to 18 feel that they hardly ever get enough sleep. In fact people from the ages of 13 to 65 habitually feel tired.

Research throughout the world has shown 7 hours of sleep is the most beneficial amount of sleep for most adults. Shockingly, we now know that 15% of young people between the ages of 12 to 18 get less than 6 hours of sleep most nights. Even more alarming, the group of 13 to 18-year-olds gets even less sleep on weekends.

This becomes a tremendous problem and burden for teenagers who need 9 to 10 hours of sleep every night. Lack of sleep interferes with their hormone production, especially their growth hormones. Lack of sleep affects their metabolism, which then makes it almost impossible for them to lose weight.

Sleep-deprived teenagers are overtired, sluggish, cranky, sullen, moody, and often doze off in class. Even worse, they sometimes doze off behind the wheel!

Many of these teens have become addicted to stimulating themselves especially with caffeine in the form of coffee, soft drinks and products such as Red Bull. Is it any wonder Starbucks has gone from 9 stores to 19,000 stores today?

Most teens today drink way too much caffeine and then they can't go to sleep at night. Many take over-the-counter pills like melatonin, or their own or parents' prescriptions like Lunesta and Ambien to help them get to sleep.

When they awaken the next morning they feel groggy, sluggish, and their thinking is fuzzy. Now they need their "fix." Stimulating drinks and food such as sugary cereal, a donut or two, or a Danish and a few cups of coffee, just to wake them up.

What a vicious cycle! These poor habits your teenager creates won't solve the problem of lack of sleep. These habits just create other problems.

A recent study of thousands of teenager worldwide ascertained that teens need a *minimum* of 9 hours of sleep every night. It was a shock to discover that only 3% of the teens in the study got 9 hours of sleep! Most teens get an average of about 6 ½ hours of sleep on school nights and even less on weekends.

Sadly, it has been established that for every hour of nightly sleep a teenager loses, there is a high – a very high – percentage that end up feeling sad, hopeless, alienated, depressed, suicidal, and often with an increased tendency toward drug usage. That's right, lack of sleep can be dangerous to your teenager's physical and *mental* health.

Teens who sleep as little as 6 hours a night display reduced or impaired brain function. This impacts their self-control, awareness of consequences, good judgment, self-confidence, and self-esteem. We know that being a teen is very often a most difficult time. However lack of sleep only amplifies those difficulties.

Parents!
Pay attention!
Is your teenager getting enough sleep?
6 hours?
Not good enough.

Remember, teenagers need at least 9 hours of sleep every night.

It's time for tough love.
Starting now at least 60 minutes before lights out, no more video games, e-readers, iPads, computers, cell phones, and yes even TV!

YIKES!

Doable?
Yes, but not easy.
It requires discipline! Yours and theirs.

Be prepared, because your teenager will probably fight you all along the way. Buy some good books, magazines, even comic books for your teenager to read before going to sleep.

Purchase the *Lights Out* Sleep Hypnosis MP3 created especially for teens. They can listen to it every night, even while reading in bed. Their *Lights*

Out Sleep Hypnosis MP3 will help them drift off to sleep. It will also help reduce stress.

It is worth it? Yes! You will see a difference in your teenager's behavior. They will see a difference in the way they feel.

But most of all, your son or daughter will not only feel better, they will look better, think better, be more active, and enjoy their life more.

Get started now, today!
It is worth it.

DO IT!

Many of the rules for helping your child get a good night's sleep are the same as the rules for an adult. These rules for a goodnight's sleep are very important.

Starting now:

Make sure your child get some physical exercise every day.

Make sure they are involved in activities where they are actually moving, not just organized sports where they may spend most of their time sitting on the bench waiting for a chance to play.

Today too many children do not get very much physical playtime at school or at home. When they get home they usually grab a snack and plop down in front of the TV, or get on a mobile device or computer, or start playing video games. It seems as though the only exercise most of our children get anymore is exercising their thumbs!

Some physical exercise after school is very important it will help them fall asleep easily at night. Physical exercise can even help them lose weight.

Make sure your child is getting exposed to sunshine every day.

Another benefit of being outside and physically active is exposure to sunshine, which will help regulate their melatonin production. Bright natural light during the day combined with a quiet, semi-dark, soothing room at night will help your child go to sleep and stay asleep.

I wonder if you have ever noticed that when your child has been outside playing at the beach, or the park, or even playing in the back yard, they tend to fall asleep quickly and sleep soundly?

So many of our children are cooped up all day at school or at home and are rarely exposed to sunlight. Make sure they get some sunshine every day.

Limit or eliminate your child's consumption of caffeine.

Today our children are exposed to many caffeinated foods and beverages, many of them on a daily basis. Think about it, colas and almost all sodas (especially Mountain Dew) are high in caffeine. Other foods containing caffeine are chocolate, many candies, iced tea, chocolate milk, chocolate ice cream, sports drinks, and of course coffee.

Caffeine has a much more powerful effect on children! Therefore for your child to sleep well, caffeine should either be eliminated, or certainly never consumed after noontime. Eliminating caffeine will enable your child (and you) to have a better night's sleep.

Your child should eat at least 3 to 4 hours before their bedtime whenever this is possible.

Research has shown that many young children eat around 7 o'clock and are in bed around 8:30 to 9:00. If you can't always have your child eat 3 or 4 hours before bedtime, then provide your children with a light, easy-to-digest meals such as poached eggs, toast, milk, sugarless cereal, bananas, etc. This will help your child to sleep without tossing, turning, and awakening during the night to go to the bathroom or even worse, having nightmares.

Create a good feeling around bedtime.

Always be careful about putting negative thoughts about sleep into your child head. Never pressure your child to sleep and never make your child feel bad if they don't get to sleep easily or that there is something wrong with them because they have a hard time sleeping.

Please don't do as I did. When my children were very little, I did some very dumb things like singing Rock-a-Bye Baby to them. It has that line, "When the bough breaks the cradle will fall, and down will come baby cradle and all."

Or teaching them the little prayer, you know the one that goes, "Now I lay me down to sleep, I pray the Lord my soul to keep, if I should *die* before I wake I pray the Lord my soul to take." Then I would turn off all lights, and shut the door, and expect them to peacefully go to sleep! What was I thinking?

That's when the call for water would start, "Mommy I need a drink," or, "I need to go potty."

Or they would sneak out of bed and stand in the hall where they would be in the light and could see mom and dad watching television. It took me a while to get it. I discovered that I could allow a small nightlight on in their room and I could leave their door open so they did not feel abandoned or cut off from their family.

Guess what!
They started staying in bed and falling asleep quickly, without all the problems associated with trying to get children to go to bed and to go to sleep. These few simple steps helped my children to create excellent sleeping habits that they still have to this day.

I am so glad that I somehow figured out what would help them to see sleep as something inviting and pleasurable, not as a punishment or something that mean adults do to their children.

I did it!
So can you.
Relax.

Begin now to teach your children to start enjoying sleep.

Snorer

Everyone knows that snoring can be a huge problem. It can interfere with sleep for the person who snores as well as the person who has to listen to the snorer.

Rule out sleep apnea.

Quite often snoring is caused by sleep apnea, a condition where the person actually stops breathing for several seconds while they are asleep. Sleep apnea can be serious, leading to reduced oxygen levels, not feeling rested, and other health issues.

Risk factors for sleep apnea include being overweight, sleeping on your back, sleeping with your mouth open, or more often from weak, flaccid throat muscles, which can also cause snoring. If you are a snorer, I urge you to check with your doctor or a sleep clinic to be tested for sleep apnea.

Sing and hum!

Recent research published in the U.K. Lancet reported that snorers have weak throat muscles. The Lancet article recommends that snorers should start humming or singing loudly for at least 20 to 30 minutes a day. Sing in the shower; sing or hum when you're alone in your car; sing when you are stuck in traffic; sing or hum when working outside in the yard; sing or hum when you work out, or go for a walk, or a run.

Snorers who participated in the study and faithfully practiced singing and humming for at least 20 to 30 minutes every day began to snore much less and felt so much more rested throughout the day.

Get those throat muscles moving. Make them strong. Sing yourself to serenity, peace, and a good night's sleep.

Lose some weight.

Losing weight will help reduce snoring especially if you are obese. Not only will you look great, you will sleep better and feel better.

Turn over on your side.

Learn to sleep on your side. Pregnant women learn to do this and so can you.

Shut your mouth! Please!

If you can breathe comfortably through your nose, consider lightly taping your mouth shut before bed, using paper surgical tape available at any drugstore. There are also chin straps to wear at night to keep you jaw in place. This will also help if you suffer from dry mouth.

Listen to your *Quiet Down* Sleep Hypnosis MP3.

It will reprogram your subconscious mind to assist you in making the above changes and also help you drift into deeper, more restful states of sleep.

Snoree

If your partner or beloved snores and keeps you awake all night, you need help. Their snoring has become *your* sleep problem.

He or she snores away while you lie wide-awake, frustrated, angry, and unable to sleep. You just lay their waiting for the next snort or snore.

You, the person being bombarded with the sounds of the snoring, need help as much as the snorer. Through hypnosis you can learn how to tune out the noise of their snoring. Believe me you *can* learn to sleep even as you partner blissfully snores on.

People who live and work in noisy environments tune out the noise of a city like New York with its unending traffic, buses, sirens, helicopters, and buildings so close to one another that people can hear their neighbors' music, TV, laughter, fighting, (and yes, even their lovemaking!) on a hot summer night. They may even hear a neighbor snoring! Yet they learn to tune out all that noise, to not be bothered by it, and to just go to sleep.

With a little help from this book and your *Tune Out a Snorer* Sleep Hypnosis MP3 you will learn how to tune out the snorer.

That's right.

Hypnosis with some guided imagery (your MP3) will teach your subconscious mind to no longer listen to or to be bothered by the sound of your partner's snoring.

This is called selective listening.

Have you ever purchased a chiming clock that chimes every hour on the hour? For the first ten days or so you wonder why you ever bought the damn clock. You hear it all night long. Then just about the time that you were ready to throw it away, you discover that you are no longer hearing it chime. You are sleeping all night. This is selective listening. The clock is still chiming but you are no longer listening for the chimes.

Starting now the sound of the snoring will become a part of your new mental imagery, your selective listening. The snoring will begin to soothe you rather than annoy you. You will incorporate the sound of the snoring into the soothing sound on your MP3.

As you listen to your *Tune Out a Snorer* Sleep Hypnosis MP3, you will be gently drifting on your little sailboat, lulled to sleep by the soothing sounds of the gentle sea. As you relax, the gentle rocking back-and-forth of your anchored boat lulls you deeper and deeper to sleep. Hear the sound of the gulls calling out to each other as they fly overhead.

Soothing sounds.
Peaceful sounds.
Lulling you to sleep.
Drifting,

Floating,
Dreaming,

Try it.
You can do it.
Let it happen.

Commit to Change

Deep, Deep Breaths

One thing I need to teach you is how to breathe.

Oh, I know that you're breathing as you read this, but I want you to learn how to do *deep* breathing. Deep breathing oxygenates your brain so that you can relax and relearn how to sleep. You always learn better when you are relaxed.

If you are like most people I work with, you probably do shallow chest breathing.

Check yourself right now. Come on. Go ahead and take a deep breath and exhale. That's right.

Did you lift your chest or your shoulders up as you inhaled? Did you quickly blow out the air in your lungs as you exhaled?

Wrong! Wrong! Not very relaxing was it?

The proper way to do deep breathing is to relax your shoulders and to not lift up your chest at all. Instead you will inflate your belly as you inhale and then suck it backwards to your spine as you exhale.

Can't quite do it? Okay, it really is quite easy once you get the hang of it. Here is how you can learn to take those deep breaths:

Get a letter-size piece of paper; anything will do.

Lie on your back on the floor or your bed and put a pillow beneath you head.

Place the piece of paper on you belly.

Inhale and lift the paper up by sticking out your belly as you breathe in thru your nose, then let the paper come back down as you open your mouth slightly and exhale very slowly.

Come on. Try it again.

Inhale, belly out.
Exhale, belly in.

See, it's easy. You did it! Relaxing isn't it?

Watch a baby sleeping and you will see they breathe this way naturally.

Try it again. Inhale, belly out. Hold it. Open your mouth slightly and then exhale very slowly, belly in.

For some of you this maybe just the opposite of how you were taught to breath, to take a deep breath by pushing your chest out and to sucking your belly in.

Do it right from now on.
Deep breathe this way for three slow breaths, at

least three times a day. You can learn how to do it. Practice makes perfect.

Putting It All Together

You have read this book; you have begun to listen to your particular Sleep Hypnosis MP3; and you have discovered that you already knew more than you thought you did.

You have also discovered some very important things that you did not know. These are the things that have been interfering with your ability to get a good night's sleep.

This time it's different.

Now you are aware and are committed to make the changes you need to make to enable you to get the kind of sleep that you long for and that you deserve.

What is different this time?
Hypnotherapy!

It's simple.
Make the commitment to read and review this book, listen to your Sleep Hypnosis MP3 every night, and write in your Sleep Journal every day. Make the commitment to do these things for at least 21 days consecutive days.

Hypnotherapy exceeds any other method that has been used to help people relearn how to sleep. This book contains all the information that you need to redirect your thinking regarding your new sleep habits.

Read your book over and over again until you have almost memorized it. Remember to highlight, underline, dog-ear the pages, and memorize those things that apply to your particular sleep problem.

Listen to your Sleep Hypnosis MP3 every night for the next three weeks. Over time it will enable you to change your negative stories, attitudes, and beliefs that have been interfering with you being able to sleep.

Learn how to breathe. I know that you know how to breathe, but I am talking about deep, deep, relaxed breathing. Follow the instructions in the previous chapter.

Every morning, for the next 21 days, write in your Sleep Journal. (See page 141.) This will help educate your subconscious mind how to reestablish your natural sleep rhythm.

Now it is time for you to get either a highlighter or a pen; as you read through the following list, check off the things you need to be committed to change.

If you really want results, don't, I repeat, DON'T ignore this section of the book!

It is very, very, important!

If you were a client in my office this would be your homework. I would have you do this and then we would go over each item at our next appointment. However since you are on your own, you have to be even more disciplined and committed to make these changes. You won't regret it!

Get ready. Check off only the following things that you need to change. Then give yourself 21 days for those changes to take place. Practice, practice, practice making the changes you need to make every day and every night. Then watch the magic begin to happen.

The following list covers most everything that interferes with most people's ability to get a good night's sleep. Which ones are you willing to change?

1. Your Bed:
If your bed is over 7 years old consider buying a new one! You can start by first getting new sheets, blankets, and pillows, and then as soon as you can afford it, buy a new bed. Also, remember always make your bed everyday and to air out your bedding once or twice a month.

2. S.O.S.:
Adults, only use your bed for sleep or sex! Nothing else.

3. Families and Beds:

Only use your bed for yourself and your mate. Your bed should not be a community gathering place.

4. Pets and Beds:

I know you love your pet, but it is time to declare your bed a pet-free zone.

5. Alcohol:

Never use alcohol to put yourself to sleep. It will! But you will awaken two or three hours later and find it difficult to go back to sleep.

6. Caffeine:

The most used stimulant worldwide is caffeine. No caffeine 6 hours before bedtime. If you must drink coffee late in the day or in the evening please drink decaf.

7. Tobacco:

Nicotine is a stimulant. Skip that last cigarette ritual before bedtime. Don't light up if you should awaken during the night. Better yet just quit smoking!

8. Full Moon:

The light of a full moon might be beautiful but block it out. You can lose 20 to 30 minutes of sleep every night when there is a full moon. Get blackout curtains or wear an eye mask.

9. Sunshine:

If you want to have a healthy sleep cycle, welcome natural light into your life every day.

10. Your clock:

Your clock is your enemy. Turn it around to face the wall. You don't need to see it during the night.

11. Too little sleep:

Sleep deprivation is dangerous. 5% of California drivers admit they have nodded off while driving.

12. Meds and beds:

Sleep is your best medicine. Check with your pharmacist or doctor to find out if your medications may be keeping you awake and if so, ask if there is an alternative.

13. Don't dine late:

What you eat and *when* you eat will always affect the quality of your sleep.

14. No pigging out:

You need at least four hours between putting down your fork and laying down your body on the sofa or the bed.

15. Foods good for sleep:

There are foods that you can eat before bedtime that will help you sleep, such as bananas, cherries, milk, yogurt, turkey, walnuts, and many, many more.

16. Exercise:

Aim for at least 30 minutes of exercise, 5 times a week. Do not exercise too close to your sleep time. However move your body every day. If you have any questions about starting an exercise program, check with your doctor.

17. Sound the alarm:
Daylight Savings always causes a spike in injuries and costly mental mistakes. Be prepared to get the extra sleep that you need in order to be rested and alert.

18. No electronics before bed:
Avoid the blue light coming from computers, mobile devices and television. Wear amber goggles if necessary. Read real books or magazines.

19. Snorer:
Lose weight and sing and hum to strengthen your throat muscles. Sleep on your side or your stomach. If you can breathe through your nose, find a way to shut your mouth. Some people find that loosely taping their mouth with a small piece of surgical tape helps.

20. Sleeping with a snorer:
Tune out! Let go of your anger. Stop waiting for the next snore. Turn on your *Tune Out a Snorer* Sleep Hypnosis MP3, listen to it, and let it put you to sleep.

21. Sleep Rituals:
Always do the same things, in the same way, and at the same time every night as you prepare yourself to go to sleep. Doing these rituals every night will educate your subconscious mind to know it's time for you to go to sleep.

22. Track your progress:

Every morning write your results in your 21-Day Sleep Journal. (See next chapter.)

Whatever problems you have checked off, go back to that particular section in this book, and read it in its entirety. Then get to work and make the changes. Do the work and sleep will begin to come easily and effortlessly.

Trust yourself, trust your subconscious mind, and trust the power of your own thoughts.

Change your thoughts.
Change your sleeping habits.

Remember to always do the same things, in the same way, and at the same time as you prepare to go to sleep.

You will sleep.
So enjoy.

YOUR 21 DAY SLEEP JOURNAL

It is very important for you to keep a Sleep Journal for the next 21 days. You will keep a brief daily record and as well as an end-of-the-week summary.

By now you have purchased and are listening to your Sleep Hypnosis MP3. You have read about all the things that can prevent a good night's sleep. I also hope that you have highlighted those things that apply to you. You are committed to change those things that, in the past, have interfered with you having a good night's sleep.

One of the things you absolutely need to do is keep this Sleep Journal for the next three weeks. It is easy. It will provide questions for you to answer.

You will write the answers to questions for each day of the week followed a few more questions at the end of each week.

Please do this. It is so very important because it will help you change your attitude regarding your sleep habits. It will also enable you to develop healthy sleep routines, and to correct habits that, in the past, have interfered with you getting a good night's sleep.

I suggest you keep your journal and a pen on the night stand by your bed. Every morning when you awaken, before getting out of bed, jot down the answers to the questions. Most questions only require a word or two. At the end of each week there are a few added questions regarding your sleep for the week. This will help you to think much more positively regarding your sleep activities. You also will be able to track your progress as you discover your own natural sleep rhythm. As you do this you will begin to feel more rested and more alert throughout the day.

You can write your answers in this book, or a notebook, or you can download a free printable version:

21-Day Sleep Journal
www.holmeshypnotherapy.com/sleepjournal

Day One:

What time did you choose for your "go to bed" time?

Approximately how much time did you need to listen to your MP3 before you fell asleep?

Total time you spent in bed?

Total hours you slept?

How would you evaluate your night's sleep?

Day Two:

What time did you choose for your "go to bed" time?

Approximately how much time did you need to listen to your MP3 before you fell asleep?

Total time you spent in bed?

Total hours you slept?

How would you evaluate your night's sleep?

Day Three:

What time did you choose for your "go to bed" time?

Approximately how much time did you need to listen to your MP3 before you fell asleep?

Total time you spent in bed?

Total hours you slept?

How would you evaluate your night's sleep?

Day Four:

What time did you choose for your "go to bed" time?

Approximately how much time did you need to listen to your MP3 before you fell asleep?

Total time you spent in bed?

Total hours you slept?

How would you evaluate your night's sleep?

Day Five:

What time did you choose for your "go to bed" time?

Approximately how much time did you need to listen to your MP3 before you fell asleep?

Total time you spent in bed?

Total hours you slept?

How would you evaluate your night's sleep?

Day Six:

What time did you choose for your "go to bed" time?

Approximately how much time did you need to listen to your MP3 before you fell asleep?

Total time you spent in bed?

Total hours you slept?

How would you evaluate your night's sleep?

Day Seven:

What time did you choose for your "go to bed" time?

Approximately how much time did you need to listen to your MP3 before you fell asleep?

Total time you spent in bed?

Total hours you slept?

How would you evaluate your night's sleep?

How many nights this week did you experience deep and restful sleep?

How many nights did you sleep just "okay"?

How many nights did you feel that you never really got into a deep level of sleep?

How many nights do you feel you hardly slept at all?

How many nights did you work on changing your negative sleep thoughts into positive sleep thoughts?

Were there any nights that you needed to take sleep medication? If so, how many nights?

WEEK TWO DAILY QUESTIONS

Day Eight:

What time did you go to bed? Was it your chosen bedtime?

Approximately how long did you need to listen to your MP3 before you fell asleep?

Did you wake up during the night?

What caused you to wake up?

How long did it take you to get back to sleep?

Did you replay your MP3?

What time did you wake up in the morning?

What time did you get out of bed?

Total hours you slept?

Total time did you spent in your bed?

How would you evaluate your night's sleep?

Day Nine:

What time did you go to bed? Was it your chosen bedtime?

Approximately how long did you need to listen to your MP3 before you fell asleep?

Did you wake up during the night?

What caused you to wake up?

How long did it take you to get back to sleep?

Did you replay your MP3?

What time did you wake up in the morning?

What time did you get out of bed?

Total hours you slept?

Total time did you spent in your bed?

How would you evaluate your night's sleep?

Day Ten:

What time did you go to bed? Was it your chosen bedtime?

Approximately how long did you need to listen to your MP3 before you fell asleep?

Did you wake up during the night?

What caused you to wake up?

How long did it take you to get back to sleep?

Did you replay your MP3?

What time did you wake up in the morning?

What time did you get out of bed?

Total hours you slept?

Total time did you spent in your bed?

How would you evaluate your night's sleep?

Day Eleven:

What time did you go to bed? Was it your chosen bedtime?

Approximately how long did you need to listen to your MP3 before you fell asleep?

Did you wake up during the night?

What caused you to wake up?

How long did it take you to get back to sleep?

Did you replay your MP3?

What time did you wake up in the morning?

What time did you get out of bed?

Total hours you slept?

Total time did you spent in your bed?

How would you evaluate your night's sleep?

Day Twelve:

What time did you go to bed? Was it your chosen bedtime?

Approximately how long did you need to listen to your MP3 before you fell asleep?

Did you wake up during the night?

What caused you to wake up?

How long did it take you to get back to sleep?

Did you replay your MP3?

What time did you wake up in the morning?

What time did you get out of bed?

Total hours you slept?

Total time did you spent in your bed?

How would you evaluate your night's sleep?

Day Thirteen:

What time did you go to bed? Was it your chosen bedtime?

Approximately how long did you need to listen to your MP3 before you fell asleep?

Did you wake up during the night?

What caused you to wake up?

How long did it take you to get back to sleep?

Did you replay your MP3?

What time did you wake up in the morning?

What time did you get out of bed?

Total hours you slept?

Total time did you spent in your bed?

How would you evaluate your night's sleep?

Day Fourteen:

What time did you go to bed? Was it your chosen bedtime?

Approximately how long did you need to listen to your MP3 before you fell asleep?

Did you wake up during the night?

What caused you to wake up?

How long did it take you to get back to sleep?

Did you replay your MP3?

What time did you wake up in the morning?

What time did you get out of bed?

Total hours you slept?

Total time did you spent in your bed?

How would you evaluate your night's sleep?

How many nights this week did you experience deep and restful sleep?

How many nights did you sleep just "okay"?

How many nights did you feel that you never really got into a deep level of sleep?

How many nights do you feel you hardly slept at all?

How many nights did you work on changing your negative sleep thoughts into positive sleep thoughts?

Were there any nights that you needed to take sleep medication? If so, how many nights?

What was the average number of hours you slept each night?

Do you consistently go to sleep at the same time now?

Do you consistently wake up around the same time?

How many nights did you listen to your MP3?

How much time did you spend each night in bed?

WEEK THREE DAILY QUESTIONS

Day Fifteen:

What time did you go to bed?

Approximately how long did you need to listen to your MP3 before you fell asleep?

Did you awaken during the night?

If you did, what caused you to awaken?

How long did it take you to get back to sleep?

Did you need to replay your MP3?

What time did you wake up in the morning?

Total hours you slept?

How much time did you spend in your bed?

How would you evaluate your night's sleep?

Day Sixteen:

What time did you go to bed?

Approximately how long did you need to listen to your MP3 before you fell asleep?

Did you awaken during the night?

If you did, what caused you to awaken?

How long did it take you to get back to sleep?

Did you need to replay your MP3?

What time did you wake up in the morning?

Total hours you slept?

How much time did you spend in your bed?

How would you evaluate your night's sleep?

Day Seventeen:

What time did you go to bed?

Approximately how long did you need to listen to your MP3 before you fell asleep?

Did you awaken during the night?

If you did, what caused you to awaken?

How long did it take you to get back to sleep?

Did you need to replay your MP3?

What time did you wake up in the morning?

Total hours you slept?

How much time did you spend in your bed?

How would you evaluate your night's sleep?

Day Eighteen:

What time did you go to bed?

Approximately how long did you need to listen to your MP3 before you fell asleep?

Did you awaken during the night?

If you did, what caused you to awaken?

How long did it take you to get back to sleep?

Did you need to replay your MP3?

What time did you wake up in the morning?

Total hours you slept?

How much time did you spend in your bed?

How would you evaluate your night's sleep?

Day Nineteen:

What time did you go to bed?

Approximately how long did you need to listen to your MP3 before you fell asleep?

Did you awaken during the night?

If you did, what caused you to awaken?

How long did it take you to get back to sleep?

Did you need to replay your MP3?

What time did you wake up in the morning?

Total hours you slept?

How much time did you spend in your bed?

How would you evaluate your night's sleep?

Day Twenty:

What time did you go to bed?

Approximately how long did you need to listen to your MP3 before you fell asleep?

Did you awaken during the night?

If you did, what caused you to awaken?

How long did it take you to get back to sleep?

Did you need to replay your MP3?

What time did you wake up in the morning?

Total hours you slept?

How much time did you spend in your bed?

How would you evaluate your night's sleep?

Day Twenty-one:

What time did you go to bed?

Approximately how long did you need to listen to your MP3 before you fell asleep?

Did you awaken during the night?

If you did, what caused you to awaken?

How long did it take you to get back to sleep?

Did you need to replay your MP3?

What time did you wake up in the morning?

Total hours you slept?

How much time did you spend in your bed?

How would you evaluate your night's sleep?

How many nights this week did you experience deep and restful sleep?

How many nights did you sleep just "okay"?

How many nights do you feel you hardly slept at all?

How many nights did you change your negative sleep thoughts into positive sleep thoughts?

Did you need to take sleep medication?

What time do you consistently go to sleep now?

What time do you consistently wake up now?

How many nights did you listen to your MP3?

How much time did you spend each night in bed?

Average hours you slept each night?

How often did you go to sleep and wake up at the same time each day?

How often have you practiced the life changes that previously interfered with your sleep?

How often did you practice deep breathing to help you relax?

After you have finished your 21-Day Sleep Journal check off any of the following that now apply to you:

- o   I now sleep better most nights.
- o   I'm sleeping throughout the night.
- o   I have more restful sleep, no more tossing and turning all night.
- o   I fall asleep easily with my Sleep Hypnosis MP3.
- o   I rarely wake up during the night.
- o   If I wake up during the night, I am able to go back to sleep easily and effortlessly.
- o   I enjoy uninterrupted sleep almost every night.

Adults:

- o   I have discovered my natural 6 to 8 hours sleep time.

Children and Teenagers:

- o   Have you discovered your natural 8 to 9 hours sleep time?

Seniors:

- o   Have you discovered your natural sleep time 5 to 6 hours with a nap?

Snorers:

- o   I am sleeping better and feel well rested.

Snorees:

- o   I am no longer listening to the Snorer.

Everyone:

- o   I am feeling more rested and relaxed every day.
- o   I don't need sleep medication any more.
- o   I have found my natural sleep rhythm and I will stick to it every night.

Soon, maybe not as soon as you would have liked, perhaps sooner than you had hoped, you will discover that you're enjoying your new way of sleeping.

You now know that you are getting the correct amount of sleep for you. When you awaken, you feel relaxed, refreshed, and look forward to the new day.

You continue listening to your Sleep Hypnosis MP3.
You are relearning how to sleep.
That is magical

ABOUT DR. WANITA

Thirty years ago at the age of 57, I was out of work and down to $800 in the bank. I was living in a bedroom at a friend's house and desperately trying to figure out how I would survive. I was told I was too old for an entry-level job and too close to retirement for a corporate job. Desperate and depressed, I asked God, the Universe, Spirit Guides, Guardian Angels, or anyone who would listen, "What shall I do? What shall I do?"

I swear 'someone' kept whispering over and over again, "HYPNOTHERAPY!"

I felt as though someone was just yanking my chain. Hypnotherapy? No one is making a living doing hypnotherapy! But the whisper was very insistent and soon I could no longer ignore it.

To quiet the nagging in my mind, I got out the yellow pages (yes, there were yellow pages in those days!) and to my surprise I discovered there was actually a hypnotherapy school. Feeling a little foolish but determined to quiet the nagging voice in my head, I called the school. A delightful lady answered the phone and agreed to send me the school's information packet. When it arrived, I looked at it and thought, *New Age, airy-fairy stuff, make a living doing this? I don't think so.* And I threw it unopened into the trash.

Two weeks later the lady from the school called and asked me if I had read the material. I lied! I said it never came.

"That's odd," she said.

"Isn't it?" I replied.

"Let me check and see if I have the right address."

Of course she did. She then agreed to send me another packet. This time I opened it. The first thing I saw was that it required $500 to start the course. Once again, I tossed the packet into the trash. After all, I only had $800 to my name.

Once again, the lady from the school called. She said a lady had cancelled her reservation and would I be interested in taking that available space? I heard myself say yes. I wondered who said that? Where did that come from? I had a feeling that someone, something, was guiding me, moving me on to a new life journey.

Desperation often makes you crazy, or courageous. So before I could change my mind, I wrote the check for $500, stuffed it in an envelope and raced to the post office. I wanted to put it in the outgoing mail before I could change my mind.

For about 24 hours, I was euphoric, filled with excitement. It did not last. Instead, I was now filled with fear, panic, and dread due to my impulsive behavior. "What the hell have I done?" I thought. "Am I crazy? I need to get that money back! I will just go there and ask for a refund."

Driving down to the school, I became even more panicked. The freeway was crowded so I began to practice out loud what I would say when I got to the school. I made up dozens of excuses and reasons why they should give me my money back. When I arrived, everyone was busy and it seemed inappropriate for me to ask for my money back at that time. So I decided that I would wait until the morning break and then go to the administration office to plead my case.

Two hours later I knew, whoever or whatever had pushed or guided me to this class knew better than I did. I never asked for my money back. That day I knew I had found my calling. It has been more than three decades and I still have a full time hypnotherapy practice. Over the years I've worked with celebrities, politicians, rock stars, children, musicians, artists, students, writers, people from every walk of life, for every problem you could imagine. I have loved every moment of it.

I also have my own hypnotherapy school where I have trained hundreds of new hypnotherapists. I work very closely with my students. At my age, I long to pass on to my students all that I have learned over these many years. I tell my students, "My clients have taught me everything I know, and I'm going to teach it all to you."

Over the years I have been written up in *Elle, Cosmopolitan, Eve, Marie Claire, The London Herald, The Los Angeles Times, Larchmont Chronicle, The Santa Monica Evening Outlook,* and even *The National Enquirer!*

I've appeared on TV's *Good Morning London*, the BBC, *The Kilroy Show* (London), KABC *Early Morning* talk show, Regis Philbin's radio talk show, and many guest-speaking engagements.

My success came at an age when most people are ready to give up or retire. Remember, it is never too late to start over.

TESTIMONIALS

I had a different kind of sleep problem. When I was 16 I could not wake up in the morning. Your hypnosis technique worked on me, in fact it worked so well that I did not like it at all! I would wake up precisely at the exact time I needed to get up to get to school, even though I would have preferred to stay in bed like I used to before I came to see you and started to fall asleep every night listening to the tapes you made for me.

You gave me a great skill. You taught me how to use my subconscious mind in the most powerful way. You taught me that I could tell myself what time I needed to wake up that I would wake up. Sometimes I would even tell myself to wake up in the middle of the night just so I could test myself, and then I would put on my tape and go right back to sleep and have a wonderful lucid dream. It always worked.

I am now 22 years old and I still use all the techniques that you taught me when I was young. It still works. I sleep well. I wake up when I need to. I always wakeup easily refreshed and rested.
So I just wanted to thank you so much.

E.M.
Los Angeles, California

I didn't know what to expect because I had never been to a hypnotherapist before and my experience with Dr. Wanita was amazing. Right now I live in Florida and she still works with me through the phone and Skype. She helped me prepare for my MCAT exam and she helped my sister overcome her fear of flying and pass her LSAT exam. I highly recommend her!"

Stephanie S.
Hollywood, Florida

My brother came to see you six months ago for a sleeping problem. I was very skeptical. I told him he was just wasting his money, hypnotherapy doesn't work. Much to my surprise he has been sleeping really great for the last six months.

I am now a believer! I would like to make an appointment to see you for my problems, but sleeping is not one of them.

Thank you, I look forward to seeing you.

George G.
Santa Monica, California

The first time I went to Dr. Wanita for hypnosis I was very skeptical. She explained what hypnotherapy is and how hypnosis can be used for many things that a person might want to change in his/her life. After the amazing changes I saw in my life, I decided I wanted to help others in the same way. Even though I am now a certified hypnotherapist, I still find myself making excuses to see her at least once a month."

Rana S.
Los Angeles, California

Contact and Ordering Info

Dr. Wanita Holmes maintains a private practice and Hypnotherapy School at Sunset Gower Studios in Hollywood, California.

She is available for individual sessions at her office or via telephone or Skype.

Email: drwanita@gmail.com

Phone: 323-817-8888 (Pacific Time)

Website: www.holmeshypnotherapy.com

Order your companion Sleep Hypnosis MP3 at:

www.holmeshypnotherapy.com/mp3s

To order books by Dr. Wanita Holmes go to
amazon.com
or
www.holmeshypnotherapy.com/books